Prescription Drugs
and Their Side Effects

Prescription Drugs and Their Side Effects
is an analysis of the 250 most frequently prescribed drugs
as tabulated by the New York State Pharmacy Board and
various other listings and tabulations.

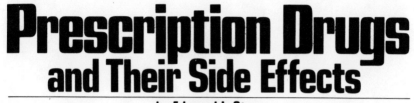

Prescription Drugs
and Their Side Effects

by Edward L. Stern

Grosset & Dunlap

Publishers — New York

Copyright © 1981, 1978, 1975 by Edward L. Stern
All rights reserved
Published simultaneously in Canada
Library of Congress catalog card number: 75-24597
ISBN 0-448-12025-9

Printed in the United States of America

1982 PRINTING

CONTENTS

Introduction

Why This Book

What prompts a layman to write a book about the side effects and adverse reactions to prescription drugs?

After all, I'm not a physician, medical researcher, pharmacist or employee of a drug company.

But I am a father. A son. A husband. I have taken prescription drugs from time to time, and I have friends and relatives who have. Most of us do.

During an eighteen-month period, individuals close to me experienced the following disturbing medical problems: My son was rushed to the hospital with a severe penicillin reaction. My mother was hospitalized after she blacked out. A cousin confided that he thought he had become impotent. And, my best friend's wife was taken off "the pill" because of an assortment of medical difficulties. In each instance, after much heartache, pain, and costly medical care, the problem was diagnosed as a reaction to a particular drug.

And so I decided to do this book to *alert* consumers to the *possible* side effects and adverse reactions of the prescription drugs they take. Side effects and reactions such as:

dizziness, dry mouth, stomach cramps, loss of balance, bleeding, fluid retention, headaches, vomiting, fever, rash, nausea, loss of appetite, itching, diarrhea, blurred vision, pains in the joints, impotence, insomnia, jitters, fluttering, constipation, shortness of breath, drowsiness, depression.

After all, if you know *in advance* the possible reactions you may encounter as a result of taking a particular drug, you'll be prepared for any health changes you experience — whether slight or pronounced — and you'll also be able to describe any unusual side effects to your own physician.

One simple example of the needless confusion, discomfort, and cost that result from taking medication without knowing all its possible effects is illustrated in the following case.

A woman I know had been taking a blood pressure medication for more than a year. During this time she was constantly bothered by a stuffy nose. She spent hundreds of dollars and many hours in doctors' offices seeking a remedy for her stuffy nose. The stuffy nose was a side effect associated with her blood pressure medication. But, unfortunately, she never connected the two. And she never mentioned the stuffy nose to the family physician who prescribed the blood pressure medication. In this age of specialization, she took her nose problem to a "nose specialist." Her discomfort probably could have been solved immediately if she had been able to connect the cause and effect to the prescription drug she was taking.

How We Determined Which Drugs to Include

A recent article in *The New York Times* estimated that more than *one billion* drug prescriptions are written by doctors in the United States each year. Chances are that you or someone in your family is taking at least one prescription drug *right now!* Just look in your medicine cabinet. If you're an average consumer, you've probably had one or more prescriptions filled in the last thirty days.

Each month, Americans purchase millions of sleeping pills, tranquilizers, diuretics, blood pressure medicines, birth control pills, decongestants, antihistamines, antidepressants, pain relievers, antibiotics, anticoagulants, weight control pills, hormones, and anticonvulsants.

We take drugs to make us feel better. To end discomfort. To stop pain. To induce sleep. To increase energy. To fight infection.

Often these drugs bring about an assortment of side effects in susceptible individuals. Since there are thousands of different prescription medicines on the market, I was faced with the problem of determining *which* drugs to include in the book and *which* to omit.

One day I was having a prescription filled at our local druggist's and noticed a large price list posted at the end of his counter. It listed the *most frequently prescribed* prescription drugs as tabulated by the New York Pharmacy Board. I had my answer. The book would include these drugs plus other popular prescription medications (250 in all) culled from various sources and would, therefore, help the greatest number of people possible without being padded with thousands of obscure drugs. My goal was to produce a volume inexpensive enough so that every consumer could afford a copy. Therefore, there may be some drugs that have been prescribed for you or your family that are *not* included in this volume. Don't be bashful. If you're concerned about the possible side effects of a drug you take that's not listed here, ask your physician to supply you with the information from his own reference material. There is a section at the end of this book for special notes. Use it to add specific information relating to your family's prescription medicines.

The intention of this book is to tell consumers . . .

1. the reason a particular drug is usually *prescribed* . . .
2. the *precautions* to observe when taking this drug . . .
3. the possible *side effects* and *adverse reactions* that may occur when taking the drug.

It should be pointed out that side effects and adverse reactions occur *only* in susceptible individuals. Most persons who take prescription drugs experience few, if any, side effects or adverse reactions. A particular drug has been prescribed because, in the opinion of the physician, the benefits far outweigh any risk.

In addition to the above, this volume also includes:

- The generic name of each drug. If your family physician will prescribe by the generic name whenever possible, you'll be able to save money on almost every prescription you fill.

- The name of the pharmaceutical company that makes the drug.

- The form the drug comes in (tablet, solution, capsule, drops, creams, etc.)

- The available strengths of the drug.

- The route for taking the drug (oral, intravaginal, rectal, intranasal, ophthalmic, etc.)

- The most commonly prescribed dosage strengths.

- An easy-to-follow A-Z index.

- Space for you and your physician to make special notes about your particular medication.

How the Information Was Compiled

With the assistance of James Molt, Ph.D., I gathered the information in three stages.

First, we edited into easy-to-understand language the information contained in the package folders sent by drug companies to physicians and pharmacists along with the drugs. Next, we verified this information, drug by drug, against the most recent *Physician's Desk Reference* (PDR), plus modifications from PDR supplements. Finally, we cross-checked all the above material against *CLIN-ALERT*, a bulletin sent to all clinics, pharmacies, and physicians to advise against any newly reported side effects, contraindications, or adverse reactions.

In researching this book, my major concern was to keep it an easy-to-use, uncomplicated reference source. Therefore, I *have not* included every possible drug form and dosage strength available for each of the 250 drugs. I have, however, listed those forms and strengths that are the most common. In addition, I have excluded, in all cases, forms of any drug that are injected since this procedure is not usually left in the hands of the consumer.

Twenty-three of the drugs appear under their generic names. These are: *Amoxicillin, Ampicillin, Chloral Hydrate, Digoxin, Erythromycin, Ferrous Sulfate, Hydrochlorothiazide, Meprobamate, Nicotinic Acid, Nitroglycerin, Papaverine HCl, Paregoric, Penicillin G Potassium, Penicillin V Potassium, Phenobarbital, Potassium Chloride, Prednisone, Propoxyphene HCl, Propoxyphene HCl compound, Quinidine Sulfate, Reserpine, Tetracycline,* and *Thyroid Tablets.* In the alphabetical listings of these twenty-three drugs we have included only the form and dosage strength that are *most frequently prescribed.* Had we tried to include every form and every strength available for each generic drug, the book would have become confusing and unwieldy since most are produced by dozens of different manufacturers in a multitude of dosage forms and strengths.

A Note on Ordering Drugs Generically:

State laws have been passed which permit a pharmacist to fill a prescription generically. Simply stated, this means that a pharmacist may stock a brand of drug which is identical to the one your physician has prescribed but less expensive. If your physician gives his permission on the prescription form, the pharmacist may substitute less expensive brands of the drug. This will occur most often if the drug is a single chemical and not a combination. For example, your physician may prescribe a specific brand of tetracycline for an infection. You take your prescription to a large pharmacy that is part of a national chain. This pharmacy carries its own brand of tetracycline which is less expensive than the brand prescribed. If your physician has indicated on the form that the prescription may be filled generically, your pharmacist is free to substitute the less expensive house brand. This results in a savings to you.

Many drugs are actually combinations of individual drugs in fixed proportions. Generally these will only be available from one pharmaceutical company. Therefore, a generic substitution is not possible. It is also possible that your physician does not wish a generic substitution even though one is possible. If he so indicates on the prescription form, your pharmacist may not make a generic substitution.

To find out if you can save money, talk with both your pharmacist and physician to determine if the prescription drug you are taking can be replaced with a less expensive brand.

A Few Words of Caution

This book is not intended to be used in any way for self-medication. Prescription drugs should be taken *only* under the supervision of a licensed physician.

In prescribing a drug, your physician is aware of the possible hazards associated with the drug and of how these may affect you. Therefore, you should *never* take any medication that has been prescribed for someone else. Various drugs affect different people in different ways.

Drugs taken in combination may produce side effects not noted when either drug is taken alone. Always inform a physician or dentist of every drug you are taking or have taken in the past. Never mix drugs unless you are so directed by a physician, and always adhere strictly to the prescribed dosage.

Most drugs are not recommended during pregnancy; pregnant women and women who plan to become pregnant should be particularly cautious, and should inform any physician treating them of their pregnancy.

The side effects and adverse reactions listed here are those the drug companies *are aware of* based upon their own research plus feedback received from physicians, pharmacists, and consumers. We have included *only the most common ones* — those that the patient, himself, can easily identify. However, just because a side effect is not listed here *does not mean that it may not be caused by the drug*. If, at any time while taking a particular medication, you experience anything abnormal, *consult your physician immediately*. It is his responsibility to determine if the side effect is tolerable in light of the therapeutic value of the drug.

In the DOSAGE section we have included many of the dosage forms available for each drug and placed an asterisk next to strengths that are contained in the New York Pharmacy List indicating *the most commonly prescribed dosage.*

Under WHEN PRESCRIBED, the common intended use for the drug (i.e., that ailment for which it is most commonly prescribed) has been listed. It may be possible that in certain cases a drug has been prescribed for some other condition or ailment. Also, since all drugs include the general phrase "Persons with known hypersensitivity to [drug name] should not use this drug," we have often omitted the phrase. For example, many drugs contain aspirin and these should be used with caution by people with known hypersensitivity to aspirin and related compounds.

The following adverse reactions have been reported in users of oral contraceptives: changes in sex drive, changes in appetite, headache, nervousness, dizziness, fatigue, backache, increase in facial hair, loss of scalp hair, skin eruptions, itching. However, an association between the symptoms and the use of oral contraceptives has been neither confirmed nor disproved. See individual entries for specific details.

In the SIDE EFFECTS AND ADVERSE REACTIONS section, the following entry appears for all antibiotics, "super-infection by nonsusceptible organism." This indicates that a particular infection may be caused by a microorganism that is immune to the action of the prescribed antibiotic. Therefore, if you do not obtain relief in a short period of time, be sure to consult your physician.

Remember, your physician is the final authority on the drug he has prescribed. His instructions, even if different from those contained in this book, should be followed.

Prescription Drugs and Their Side Effects was written for you. Your family. Your friends. It was written for you to use. To help you know what changes *may* be taking place in your own mind and body. To enable you to ask your physician intelligent questions and to *explain* certain symptoms more clearly. It is not a book for doctors or pharmacists. It is not intended to be an encyclopedia listing every conceivable side effect. It was not developed as a pharmacological tome or as the last word in drug information. Every individual is different, and drugs affect people in different ways. It is, however, designed to be an easy-to-follow, basic reference source for consumers written in easy-to-understand language. Listing each of the 250 drugs in alphabetical order, the book is intentionally devoid of subjective text material. There is no attempt to *evaluate* any drug listed.

A Note to the Reader: An asterisk placed next to a dosage strength indicates the most commonly prescribed dosage according to the New York State Pharmacy List.

ACHROMYCIN® V (Lederle Laboratories)

Generic Name: Tetracycline HCl

Dosage Form	Strength	Route
Capsule	100 mg	Oral
	250 mg*	Oral
	500 mg	Oral
Syrup	125 mg/5 cc	Oral

When Prescribed: Achromycin is an effective antibiotic prescribed for many different types of infection. It is often used in place of penicillin in patients allergic to penicillin. The length of therapy depends on the type of ailment being treated.

Precautions and Warnings: Achromycin should not be taken by persons overly sensitive to tetracycline. Not recommended for pregnant women, infants or children under the age of 8.

Side Effects and Adverse Reactions: Exaggerated sunburn can occur while taking this drug. As with other antibiotics, organisms that are not susceptible to its actions may grow. This is known as super-infection. If this occurs, the use of Achromycin should be discontinued. The following adverse reactions have been reported: loss of appetite, nausea, vomiting, diarrhea, inflammation of the tongue, difficulty swallowing, stomachache, inflammation of bowel and genital region, skin rash, hives, swelling, shock, discoloration of growing teeth.

ACTIFED—(Continued)

tion, nervousness, unsteadiness, blurred vision, double vision, ringing in ears, hallucinations, convulsions.

ACTIFED® (Burroughs Wellcome Company)

Generic Name: Triprolidine Hydrochloride, Pseudoephedrine Hydrochloride

Dosage Form	Strength	Route
Tablet	Available in one strength only	Oral
Syrup	Available in one strength only	Oral

When Prescribed: Actifed is a combination of drugs, an antihistamine and a decongestant which reduces secretions in the respiratory tract while also expanding the air passages in the lungs. This combination aids breathing in people with "hay fever" and other forms of allergy. Although it may also be prescribed for relief of symptoms of the common cold, substantial evidence for effectiveness in this area is still lacking.

Precautions and Warnings: Should be used with caution by patients with high blood pressure. A low incidence of drowsiness has been reported. Therefore, Actifed should not be taken before undertaking a task requiring complete mental alertness.

Side Effects and Adverse Reactions: Stimulation, sedation, sleepiness, dizziness, disturbed coordination, hives, rash, excessive perspiration, sensitivity to light, chills, dryness of mouth (or nose or throat), headache, fluttering of heart, thickening of bronchial secretions, tightness in chest, wheezing, nasal stuffiness, heartburn, loss of appetite, nausea, vomiting, diarrhea, constipation, difficulty in urination, menstrual irregularities, depression, fatigue, confusion, restlessness, excita-

ACTIFED–C® EXPECTORANT
(Burroughs Wellcome Company)

Generic Name: Codeine phosphate, Triprolidine Hydrochloride, Glyceryl guaiacolate, pseudoephedrine hydrochloride

Dosage Form	Strength	Route
Liquid	Available in one strength only	Oral

When Prescribed: Actifed–C Expectorant is prescribed for the relief of cough in conditions such as the common cold, acute bronchitis, asthma, breathing difficulties (croup) and emphysema.

Precautions and Warnings: Should be used with caution in patients with high blood pressure. A low incidence of drowsiness has been reported. Therefore Actifed–C Expectorant should not be taken before undertaking a task requiring complete alertness. Actifed–C Expectorant contains codeine, which may be habit forming.

Side Effects and Adverse Reactions: Mild stimulation, mild sedation (drowsiness).

AFRIN® (Schering Corporation)

Generic Name: Oxymetazoline hydrochloride

Dosage Form	Strength	Route
Spray	0.05%	Intranasal spray
Liquid	0.05%	Intranasal drops

When Prescribed: Afrin is prescribed for the relief of nasal congestion in a wide variety of allergies and infections.

Precautions and Warnings: Afrin should be used with caution by patients with high blood pressure, heart disease, overactive thyroid glands or diabetes, and by pregnant women. Children under 6 years should not use Afrin.

Side Effects and Adverse Reactions: Burning, stinging and drying of the inside of the nose; sneezing, headache, light-headedness, insomnia, heart flutters. Prolonged use of Afrin may result in what is known as "rebound" congestion, which is a "stuffy feeling" occurring after the use of the drug has ceased.

Note: This drug may now be purchased without a prescription.

ALDACTAZIDE® (Searle and Company)

Generic Name: Spironolactone with hydrochlorothiazide

Dosage Form	Strength	Route
Tablet	Available in one strength only	Oral

When Prescribed: Aldactazide is prescribed for treatment of high blood pressure, water accumulation due to congestive heart failure, cirrhosis of the liver, kidney disease and water retention of unknown cause. This preparation is a combination of two drugs which help the kidneys to pass water and salt, and relax small arteries, and help reduce the symptoms of the above-mentioned conditions. Aldactazide is usually not prescribed initially, but only after your physician has determined that the fixed combination of drugs will be proper for you.

Precautions and Warnings: This is a potent drug which requires close supervision by your physician. Your physician should be consulted if any of the symptoms listed below appears.

Side Effects and Adverse Reactions: Dryness of mouth, thirst, drowsiness, tiredness, mental confusion, diarrhea, intestinal cramps, development of breasts in males, loss of sexual drive, masculinizing traits in females (including beard growth, deepening of voice and menstrual irregularities), headache, skin eruptions, hives, fever, loss of balance, abnormal bruising, loss of appetite, nausea, vomiting, rash, itching, abnormal skin sensation (including tingling, crawling and burning), yellowing of skin, yellow appearance of

ALDACTONE® (Searle and Company)

Generic Name: Spironolactone

Dosage Form	Strength	Route
Tablet	25 mg	Oral

When Prescribed: Aldactone causes increased amounts of sodium and water to be passed from the body (diuresis). It is prescribed to lower blood pressure. It can also be prescribed for water accumulation resistant to other diuretic therapy. Aldactone is one of the constituents in Aldactazide (see previous entry) and is used to treat the same symptoms. Your physician has determined which of these drugs (Aldactone or Aldactazide) is best for your particular case.

Precautions and Warnings: Your physician should be consulted if any of the symptoms listed below appears.

Side Effects and Adverse Reactions: Dryness of mouth, thirst, drowsiness, tiredness, mental confusion, headache, diarrhea, intestinal cramps, development of breasts in males, loss of sexual drive, masculinizing traits in females (including beard growth, deepening of the voice and menstrual irregularities), skin eruptions, hives, fever, loss of balance.

Aldactazide (Continued)

objects (yellow vision), increased reactivity to sunlight, muscle spasms, weakness and restlessness, sore throat, sores in the mouth.

ALDOMET® (Merck Sharp and Dohme)

Generic Name: Methyldopa

Dosage Form	Strength	Route
Tablet	125 mg	Oral
	250 mg*	Oral
	500 mg	Oral

When Prescribed: Aldomet is usually prescribed for lowering blood pressure in patients with sustained moderate to severe high blood pressure (hypertension). Unlike most drugs which lower blood pressure, Aldomet exerts its action via the nervous system.

Precautions and Warnings: Aldomet is a potent drug that is not recommended for mild cases of high blood pressure.

Side Effects and Adverse Reactions: Sedation, headache and weakness. Lowering of blood pressure (the intended effect of the drug) may cause dizziness, light-headedness and fainting. Other adverse reactions include slowing of the heart, nasal congestion, dryness of the mouth, constipation, gas, diarrhea, nausea, vomiting, sore tongue, blackening of tongue, swollen glands in neck, weight gain, water retention, breast enlargement, lactation, impotence, loss of sexual drive, skin rash, pain in joints and muscles, skin discomfort, shaking or tremors, nightmares, mental depression, darkening of urine after voiding, fever.

ALDORIL® (Merck Sharp and Dohme)

Generic Name: Methyldopa, hydrochlorothiazide

Dosage Form	Strength	Route
Tablet	15 mg	Oral
	25 mg*	Oral

When Prescribed: Aldoril is a combination of two drugs prescribed for the control of high blood pressure especially in cases where water and salt retention is a problem. Aldoril is usually not prescribed initially after a diagnosis of high blood pressure but only when your physician has determined that the fixed combination of drugs in Aldoril is the proper dosage for you.

Precautions and Warnings: Aldoril is a potent drug which should only be taken under close supervision of your physician. Periodic blood and other tests will be done while taking Aldoril. Mothers should not nurse while taking Aldoril.

Side Effects and Adverse Reactions: Sleepiness, headache, weakness, dizziness, lightheadedness, numbness or tingling of skin, tremors, spasms, nightmares, depression, nausea, vomiting, constipation, gas, diarrhea, dryness of mouth, blackened tongue, fever, nasal congestion, breast enlargement, impotence, decreased sex drive, rash, loss of appetite, stomach irritation, cramps, blurred vision, slowing of heart rate, dryness of mouth, weight gain, water retention, skin discomfort, shaking or tremors, nightmares, depression, soreness of tongue.

AMBENYL® EXPECTORANT
(Marion Laboratories, Inc.)

Generic Name: Codeine sulfate, bromodiphenhydramine hydrochloride, diphenhydramine hydrochloride, ammonium chloride, potassium guaiacolsulfonate, menthol, alcohol

Dosage Form	Strength	Route
Liquid	Available in one strength only	Oral

When Prescribed: Ambenyl is prescribed for coughs accompanying colds and coughs accompanying allergies. The main effects of the drug are (1) reduction of frequency of coughing, (2) thinning of mucus for easier expectoration (passing from respiratory tract), (3) increase in size of bronchial tubes in lungs and (4) decrease in bronchial congestion.

Precautions and Warnings: Ambenyl causes drowsiness in some people. Patients who become drowsy should not drive vehicles or engage in activities requiring alert responses. Sleeping pills, sedatives, alcohol or tranquilizers should not be used with Ambenyl. Ambenyl contains codeine which may be habit forming. This drug may inhibit milk production in nursing mothers.

Side Effects and Adverse Reactions: Dry mouth, blurring of vision, thirst, dizziness, drowsiness, confusion, nervousness, restlessness, nausea, vomiting, diarrhea, double vision, blurring of vision, tingling, heaviness, weakness of hands, tightening of chest, difficulty in urination, constipation, nasal stuffiness, fluttering of heart, headache, in-

AMCILL® (Parke, Davis and Company)

Generic Name: Ampicillin trihydrate

Dosage Form	Strength	Route
Capsule	250 mg*	Oral
	500 mg	Oral
Chewable tablet	125 mg	Oral
Liquid	125 mg/5 ml	Oral
	250 mg/5 ml	Oral
Pediatric drops (liquid)	100 mg/1 ml	Oral

When Prescribed: Amcill is a synthetic penicillin that is effective in a wide variety of infections.

Precautions and Warnings: Amcill should not be taken by people who are allergic to penicillin. The use of any penicillin should be discontinued and your physician notified if any of the side effects or reactions listed below appear.

Side Effects and Adverse Reactions: Nausea, vomiting, chest or stomach pains, diarrhea, blackening of tongue, skin rash, hives, chills, fever, swelling, pain in joints, fainting, super-infection by nonsusceptible organisms, anemia, bruising, indigestion, darkening of the urine.

Ambenyl Expectorant (Continued)

somnia, hives, rash, increased sensitivity to sunlight, low blood pressure, heartburn.

AMOXICILLIN: The generic name for a drug produced by numerous companies in various forms and strengths. Also marketed as:
AMOXIL, Beecham;
LAROTID, Roche;
POLYMOX, Bristol;
TRIMOX, Squibb;
WYMOX, Wyeth.

Generic Name: Amoxicillin

Dosage Form	Strength	Route
Capsule	250 mg	Oral

When Prescribed: Amoxicillin is a synthetic penicillin that is prescribed for a wide variety of infections.

Precautions and Warnings: Amoxicillin should not be taken by people who are allergic to penicillin. The use of any penicillin should be discontinued and your physician notified if any of the side effects or reactions listed below appear.

Side Effects and Adverse Reactions: Nausea, vomiting, chest or stomach pains, diarrhea, skin rash, hives, chills, fever, swelling, pain in joints, fainting, super-infection by nonsusceptible organisms, anemia, bruising, indigestion, difficulty in breathing, wheezing.

AMOXIL® (Beecham Laboratories)

Generic Name: Amoxicillin

Dosage Form	Strength	Route
Capsule	250 mg	Oral
	500 mg	Oral
Liquid	125 mg/5 ml	Oral
	250 mg/5 ml	Oral
Liquid (pediatric drops)	50 mg/ml	Oral

When Prescribed: Amoxil is a synthetic penicillin that is prescribed for a wide variety of infections.

Precautions and Warnings: Amoxil should not be taken by people who are allergic to penicillin. The use of any penicillin should be discontinued and your physician notified if any of the side effects or reactions listed below appear.

Side Effects and Adverse Reactions: Nausea, vomiting, chest or stomach pains, diarrhea, skin rash, hives, chills, fever, swelling, pains in joints, fainting, super-infection by nonsusceptible organisms, anemia, bruising, indigestion.

AMPICILLIN The generic name for a drug produced by numerous companies in various forms and strengths. Also marketed as:
AMCILL®, Parke, Davis;
PENBRITEN®, Ayerst;
OMNIPEN®, Wyeth;
PEN–A®, Pfizer;
POLYCILLIN®, Bristol.

Generic Name: Ampicillin trihydrate

Dosage Form	Strength	Route
Capsule	250 mg*	Oral
	500 mg	Oral
Suspension	125 mg/5 cc	Oral
(liquid)	250 mg/5 cc	Oral

When Prescribed: Ampicillin is a synthetic penicillin that is effective in a wide variety of infections.

Precautions and Warnings: Ampicillin should not be taken by people who are allergic to penicillin. The use of any penicillin should be discontinued and your physician notified if any of the side effects or reactions listed below appear.

Side Effects and Adverse Reactions: Nausea, vomiting, chest or stomach pains, diarrhea, blackening of tongue, skin rash, hives, chills, fever, swelling, pain in joints, fainting, super-infection by nonsusceptible organisms, anemia, bruising, indigestion.

ANTIVERT® (Roerig)

Generic Name: Meclizine HCl

Dosage Form	Strength	Route
Tablet	12.5 mg*	Oral
	25 mg	Oral
Tablet	25 mg	Oral
(chewable)		

When Prescribed: Antivert is an antihistamine which has been shown to be effective in the management of nausea, vomiting, and dizziness associated with motion sickness. It is possibly effective, though not proven, in management of dizziness associated with diseases of the vestibular (balance) system.

Precautions and Warnings: Antivert is not recommended during pregnancy or for women who may become pregnant while taking the drug, nor is it recommended for preadolescent children. Because drowsiness may occur on occasion, patients should not drive cars or operate dangerous machinery.

Side Effects and Adverse Reactions: Drowsiness, dry mouth and, on rare occasions, blurred vision.

ANUSOL-HC (Parke-Davis)

Generic Name: Hydrocortisone acetate, Bismuth subgallate, Bismuth resorcin compound, Benzyl benzoate, Peruvian balsam, Zinc oxide

Dosage Form	Strength	Route
Suppository	Available in one strength only	Rectal
Cream	Available in one strength only	Rectal

When Prescribed: Anusol-HC is prescribed for the relief of pain and discomfort of hemorrhoids and other disorders of the rectal area.

Precautions and Warnings: The safe use of topical steroids during pregnancy has not been established. Anusol-HC should not be used on extensive areas or for prolonged periods of time in pregnant women.

Side Effects and Adverse Reactions: Local irritation.

APRESOLINE® (Ciba Pharmaceutical Company)

Generic Name: Hydralazine hydrochloride

Dosage Form	Strength	Route
Tablet	10 mg	Oral
	25 mg	Oral
	50 mg	Oral
	100 mg	Oral

When Prescribed: Apresoline is prescribed to reduce blood pressure in patients with high blood pressure.

Precautions and Warnings: Apresoline is a potent drug. Patients using this drug should be closely monitored by their physician. Not recommended during pregnancy.

Side Effects and Adverse Reactions: Headache, heart flutters and rapid heart rate, loss of appetite, nausea, vomiting, diarrhea, chest pains, nasal congestion, flushing, watery eyes, eye irritation, pain, numbness, or tingling in extremities, swelling, dizziness, tremors, muscle cramps, depression, disorientation, anxiety, rash, itching, fever, chills, pain in joints, constipation, difficulty in urination, breathing difficulties.

ARISTOCORT® (Lederle Laboratories)

Generic Name: Triamcinolone acetonide

Dosage Form	Strength	Route
Cream	0.025% 0.1* 0.5	Topical (apply directly to affected area)
Ointment	0.1 0.5	Topical (apply directly to affected area)
Gel	0.1%	Topical (apply directly to affected area)

Note: Also available in tablet and syrup.

When Prescribed: Aristocort is a topical steroid which reduces inflammation, itching, and swelling associated with skin disorders.

Precautions and Warnings: Aristocort is not for use in the eye. This preparation should not be used in large quantities or for extended periods of time on pregnant women.

Side Effects and Adverse Reactions: Burning sensation, itching, irritation, infected hair follicles, dryness, increased hair growth, acne, loss of pigment, skin damage.

ARTANE® (Lederle Laboratories)

Generic Name: Trihexyphenidyl HCl

Dosage Form	Strength	Route
Tablet	2 mg	Oral
	5 mg	Oral
Liquid	2 mg/5 ml	Oral
Capsule (Time Release)	5 mg	Oral

When Prescribed: Artane is prescribed to treat tremors and shaking in patients with Parkinson's disease and certain other nervous system disorders. Artane may also be prescribed to control tremors caused by other drugs.

Precautions and Warnings: Artane therapy is usually prolonged. Frequent physical and eye examinations are necessary.

Side Effects and Adverse Reactions: Dryness of mouth, blurring of vision, dizziness, nausea, nervousness, skin rash, delusions, hallucinations, mental confusion, vomiting, agitation, constipation, drowsiness, urinary difficulties, rapid heart beat, weakness, headache.

ATARAX® (Roerig)

Generic Name: Hydroxyzine HCl, alcohol (liquid only)

Dosage Form	Strength	Route
Tablet	10 mg	Oral
	25 mg*	Oral
	50 mg	Oral
	100 mg	Oral
Liquid	Available in one strength only	Oral

When Prescribed: Atarax is prescribed for a wide variety of conditions in which anxiety, tension, and emotional stress are apparent. It is effective in controlling vomiting in stressful situations.

Precautions and Warnings: Atarax should not be taken with alcohol, sedatives, sleeping pills or tranquilizers unless specifically directed by your physician. If drowsiness occurs you should not drive or operate dangerous machinery. Atarax should not be taken by nursing mothers.

Side Effects and Adverse Reactions: Drowsiness, dryness of mouth, tremor, convulsions.

ATIVAN (Wyeth Laboratories)

Generic Name: Lorazepam

Dosage Form	Strength	Route
Tablet	0.5 mg	Oral
	1.0 mg	Oral
	2.0 mg	Oral

When Prescribed: Ativan is prescribed for relief of the anxiety, tension, agitation, irritability, and insomnia associated with certain emotional or physical disorders.

Precautions and Warnings: This drug should not be taken with sedatives, sleeping pills, or alcohol. Patients who use Ativan should not drive or operate dangerous machinery. Abrupt cessation of this drug after prolonged use may cause withdrawal symptoms. Ativan should not be used by children under 12, by pregnant woman in the first three months of pregnancy, nor by nursing mothers.

Side Effects and Adverse Reactions: Sedation, dizziness, weakness, unsteadiness, disorientation, depression, nausea, changes in appetite, headache, sleep disturbance, agitation, skin problems, visual problems, gastrointestinal upset.

ATROMID–S® (Ayerst Laboratories)

Generic Name: Clofibrate

Dosage Form	Strength	Route
Capsule	500 mg*	Oral

When Prescribed: Atromid–S, along with proper diet and other measures, is used to reduce elevated cholesterol and/or fat levels in the blood. It is also used for treatment of people with fatty subcutaneous masses resulting from high fat levels in the blood.

Precautions and Warnings: Should not be taken by pregnant women or nursing mothers. In women who plan to become pregnant, Atromid–S should be withdrawn several months before conception.

Side Effects and Adverse Reactions: Nausea, diarrhea, abdominal distress, muscle cramping, aching, weakness, pains in joints, fatigue, drowsiness, dizziness, headache, increased appetite, weight gain, "flu-like" symptoms, decreased sex drive, impotence, vomiting, flatulence, skin rash, loss of hair, dry skin, hives, itching, heart flutters, chest pains.

AURALGAN® OTIC SOLUTION
(Ayerst Laboratories)

Generic Name: Antipyrine, benzocaine, glycerin dehydrated, oxyquinoline sulfate

Dosage Form	Strength	Route
Liquid	Available in one strength only	Otic (ear) drops

When Prescribed: Auralgan is prescribed for the relief of pain and the reduction of inflammation in middle-ear infections. It is often used in conjunction with antibiotics. Auralgan is also used to facilitate the removal of ear wax.

Precautions and Warnings: Should not be used by individuals who are sensitive to benzocaine.

Side Effects and Adverse Reactions: No adverse reactions to properly administered Auralgan have been reported.

AVC CREAM (Merrell-National Laboratories)

Generic Name: Sulfanilamide, Aminacrine hydrochloride, Allantoin

Dosage Form	Strength	Route
Cream	4-oz. tube	Intravaginal
Suppository	16/box	Intravaginal

When Prescribed: AVC Cream is prescribed for the relief of symptoms caused by infections of the vagina. Symptomatic improvements usually occur in a few days, but treatment is normally continued through one complete menstrual cycle.

Precautions and Warnings: AVC Cream should not be used by patients overly sensitive to sulfonamides, or if any of the adverse reactions listed below occur.

Side Effects and Adverse Reactions: Local discomfort, burning sensation, superinfection by nonsusceptible organisms.

AZO GANTANOL® (Roche Laboratories)

Generic Name: Sulfamethoxazole, phenazopyridine hydrochloride

Dosage Form	Strength	Route
Tablet	Available in one strength only	Oral

When Prescribed: Azo Gantanol is prescribed for urinary tract infections, primarily of the kidney and the bladder, in which pain is a complicating factor and in which no urinary obstruction is present.

Precautions and Warnings: Azo Gantanol is usually not prescribed for children under 12, nor for pregnant women at term or nursing mothers. It should not be taken by people sensitive to sulfonamides. Should be taken with adequate fluid intake. The red-orange color of the urine after taking this medication is normal.

Side Effects and Adverse Reactions: Easy bruising, slow clotting of blood, cuts that do not heal, sore throat, fever, sores in the mouth, generalized skin eruptions, hives, skin peeling, itching, swollen eyes, fainting, joint pain, nausea, vomiting, abdominal pains, diarrhea, lack of appetite, headache, pain in the extremities, mental depression, convulsions, loss of balance, hallucinations, ringing in the ears, dizziness, insomnia, fever, chills, frequent urination, lack of urination, super-infection by nonsusceptible organisms.

AZO GANTRISIN® (Roche Laboratories)

Generic Name: Sulfisoxazole, phenazopyridine hydrochloride

Dosage Form	Strength	Route
Tablet	Available in one strength only	Oral

Note: Azo Gantrisin is similar to Azo Gantanol in that both contain a form of sulfonamide and the same pain reliever. Azo Gantrisin is faster acting but does not produce as high a level of active bacterial effectiveness.

When Prescribed: See Azo Gantanol.

Precautions and Warnings: See Azo Gantanol.

Side Effects and Adverse Reactions: See Azo Gantanol.

BACTRIM DS (Roche Laboratories)

Generic Name: Trimethoprim, Sulfamethoxazole

Dosage Form	Strength	Route
Tablet	Double strength	Oral
Tablet	Regular strength	Oral
Liquid	Available in one strength only	Oral
Pediatric liquid	Available in one strength only	Oral

When Prescribed: Bactrim DS is a combination of drugs prescribed for the treatment of certain infections.

Precautions and Warnings: Bactrim DS is not recommended during pregnancy or for nursing mothers. If any of the side effects or adverse reactions listed below appear, consult your physician.

Side Effects and Adverse Reactions: Rash, sore throat, stomach upset, nausea, vomiting, abdominal pains, diarrhea, yellowing of skin, headache, body aches, depression, convulsions, hallucinations, ringing in the ears, dizziness, loss of balance, insomnia, apathy, fatigue, weakness, nervousness, fever, chills, urinary difficulties.

BENADRYL® (Parke, Davis and Company)

Generic Name: Diphenhydramine hydrochloride

Dosage Form	Strength	Route
Liquid (Elixir)	12.5 mg/5 cc	Oral
Capsule	25 mg	Oral
	50 mg	Oral

When Prescribed: Benadryl, an antihistamine, is prescribed for hay fever, nasal congestion, conjunctivitis (pinkeye) due to allergy, mild forms of hives and swelling due to allergy, prevention of reactions due to transfusions of blood or plasma, hypersensitivity of skin due to allergy. Benadryl is also effective in the prevention and control of motion sickness. Benadryl is often prescribed for patients with mild forms of Parkinson's disease or for patients with Parkinson's disease who are unable to tolerate more potent drugs.

Precautions and Warnings: Benadryl should not be taken with alcohol, sedatives, sleeping pills or tranquilizers. Drowsiness is possible with Benadryl; therefore patients should refrain from activities requiring mental alertness such as driving a car or operating dangerous machinery. Should not be taken by nursing mothers.

Side Effects and Adverse Reactions: Drowsiness, confusion, nervousness, restlessness, nausea, vomiting, diarrhea, blurring of vision, double vision, difficulty in urination, constipation, nasal stuffiness, loss of balance, heart flutters, headache, insomnia, rash, hives, heartburn, tightness of chest, wheezing, dryness of mouth, nose, throat, excessive perspiration, chills,

BENADRYL® ELIXIR (Parke-Davis and Company)

Generic Name: Diphenhydramine hydrochloride, alcohol

Dosage Form	Strength	Route
Liquid	12.5 mg/5 cc	Oral

When Prescribed: Benadryl Elixir is prescribed for the same disorders as Benadryl. The elixir contains the same active compound as Benadryl, with the addition of alcohol.

Precautions and Warnings: See Benadryl.

Side Effects and Adverse Reactions: See Benadryl.

Benadryl (Continued)

sensitivity to sunlight, dizziness, disturbed coordination, euphoria, ringing in the ears, loss of appetite, change in menstrual cycle, thickening of bronchial secretions, convulsions.

BENDECTIN® (Merrell-National Laboratories)

Generic Names: Doxylamine succinate, pyridoxine hydrochloride

Dosage Form	Strength	Route
Tablet	Available in one strength only	Oral

When Prescribed: Bendectin is for the control of vomiting and nausea associated with pregnancy (morning sickness). It also contains vitamin B6, which may be deficient during pregnancy. Bendectin is coated so that a dose taken at bedtime will be effective in the morning hours when most needed. Bendectin may also be prescribed for severe daytime nausea associated with pregnancy.

Precautions and Warnings: If drowsiness occurs, patients should not undertake dangerous tasks such as driving or operating machinery.

Side Effects and Adverse Reactions: Headache, drowsiness, nervousness, heartburn, fluttering of heart, diarrhea, disorientation, irritability, loss of balance.

BENEMID® (Merck Sharp and Dohme)

Generic Name: Probenecid

Dosage Form	Strength	Route
Tablet	Available in one strength only	Oral

When Prescribed: Benemid is prescribed for people with gout and gouty arthritis. It helps the kidneys to clear the body of uric acid. It is also prescribed for use in patients who are receiving various types of penicillin. Benemid helps elevate and prolong the effective concentration of penicillin in the body.

Precautions and Warnings: Benemid should not be taken with aspirin or any pain relievers containing salicylates as these will greatly reduce the effectiveness of Benemid. It is not usually prescribed for children under 2 years of age.

Side Effects and Adverse Reactions: Headache, loss of appetite, nausea, vomiting, frequent urination, fainting, skin rash, itching, fever, sore gums, flushing, dizziness, anemia.

BENTYL® (Merrell-National Laboratories)

Generic Name: Dicyclomine hydrochloride

Dosage Form	Strength	Route
Capsule	Available in one strength only	Oral
Tablet	Available in one strength only	Oral
Syrup	Available in one strength only	Oral

When Prescribed: Bentyl is prescribed for the treatment of peptic ulcer. It acts by reducing muscle spasm in the gastrointestinal tract. Bentyl may also be useful in other gastrointestinal disorders. The syrup is often prescribed for the treatment of colic in infants.

Precautions and Warnings: If this drug produces drowsiness or blurred vision you should not drive or operate dangerous machinery. This drug may decrease sweating which can lead to heat prostration in hot environments.

Side Effects and Adverse Reactions: Dry mouth, urinary difficulties, blurred vision, rapid heart beat, heart flutters, visual disturbances, loss of taste, headache, nervousness, drowsiness, weakness, dizziness, insomnia, nausea, vomiting, impotence, suppression of lactation in nursing mothers, constipation, bloated feeling, rash, mental confusion or excitement (especially in older persons), decreased sweating, muscle or skeletal pain.

BENTYL® with PHENOBARBITAL (Merrell-National Laboratories)

Generic Name: Dicyclomine hydrochloride phenobarbital, (alcohol in syrup)

Dosage Form	Strength	Route
Capsule	Available in one strength only	Oral
Tablet	Available in one strength only	Oral
Syrup	Available in one strength only	Oral

When Prescribed: Bentyl is prescribed for the treatment of peptic ulcer and may also be useful in the treatment of other gastrointestinal disorders. The syrup is often prescribed for the treatment of colic in infants. In addition to a drug which reduces gastrointestinal muscle spasms, this preparation contains phenobarbital which is a sedative.

Precautions and Warnings: Phenobarbital may be habit forming. If this drug produces drowsiness or blurred vision you should not drive or operate dangerous machinery. This drug may decrease sweating which can lead to heat prostration in hot environments.

Side Effects and Adverse Reactions: Dry mouth, urinary difficulties, blurred vision, rapid heart beat, heart flutters, visual disturbances, loss of taste, headache, nervousness, drowsiness, weakness, dizziness, insomnia, nausea, vomiting, impotence, suppression of lactation in nursing mothers, constipation, bloated feeling, rash, mental confusion and/or excitement (especially in older persons), decreased sweating, muscle or skeletal pain.

BENYLIN® COUGH SYRUP
(Parke, Davis and Company)

Generic Name: Diphenhydramine hydrochloride, ammonium chloride, sodium citrate, chloroform, menthol, alcohol

Dosage Form	Strength	Route
Liquid	Available in one strength only	Oral

When Prescribed: For patients with colds or allergies Benylin, an antihistamine, is prescribed as a cough suppressant.

Precautions and Warnings: Should not be taken with sleeping pills, sedatives, alcohol or tranquilizers. If drowsiness occurs, patients should not operate motor vehicles or machinery. Benylin may inhibit lactation in nursing mothers.

Side Effects and Adverse Reactions: Drowsiness, confusion, nervousness, restlessness, nausea, vomiting, diarrhea, blurring of vision, double vision, difficulty in urination, constipation, nasal stuffiness, dizziness, heart flutters, headache, insomnia, hives, rash, increased sensitivity to sunlight, low blood pressure, heartburn, tightness in chest, wheezing, dryness of mouth, nose, throat, tingling, heaviness, weakness of hands, thickening of secretions from chest, ringing in the ears, convulsions, hysteria, loss of appetite, changes in menstrual pattern, tightness of chest, disturbed coordination, excitation, irritability, tremors.

BRETHINE (Geigy Pharmaceuticals)

Generic Name: Terbutaline sulfate

Dosage Form	Strength	Route
Tablet	5.0 mg	Oral
	2.5 mg	Oral

When Prescribed: Brethine is prescribed for aiding breathing in patients with asthma, bronchitis, or emphysema.

Precautions and Warnings: This drug should not be used by children under 12 years old.

Side Effects and Adverse Reactions: Nervousness, tremors, headache, rapid heart beat, heart flutters, drowsiness, nausea, vomiting, sweating, muscle cramps.

BUTAZOLIDIN® (Geigy Pharmaceuticals)

Generic Name: Phenylbutazone

Dosage Form	Strength	Route
Tablet	Available in one strength only	Oral

When Prescribed: Butazolidin is a potent drug prescribed for the relief of pain and inflammation of gout, various forms of arthritis, and other disorders of muscle and bone characterized by pain and inflammation.

Precautions and Warnings: Butazolidin is not considered a simple pain reliever and is never prescribed casually. A patient using this drug should be examined often by his/her physician. Adverse reactions can occur rapidly; therefore the patient should immediately report anything abnormal to his physician. Patients should not drive or operate machinery. Should be taken immediately before or after meals or with milk to minimize gastric irritation.

Note: Rarely used in children under fourteen years and in senile patients.

Side Effects and Adverse Reactions: Fever, sore throat, sores in the mouth, indigestion, heartburn, slow-healing cuts, blood which does not clot, easy bruising, dark or bloody stools, significant weight gain, water retention with swelling, stomach or intestinal cramps or pain, nausea, vomiting, diarrhea, bloating, swollen glands, hepatitis, purple spots on skin, itching, general skin eruptions, hives, pains in joints, fever, rash, blood in the urine, frequent urination, lack of urination,

BUTAZOLIDIN® ALKA (Geigy Pharmaceuticals)

Generic Name: Phenylbutazone, dried aluminum hydroxide gel, magnesium trisilicate

Dosage Form	Strength	Route
Capsule	Available in one strength only	Oral

Note: Butazolidin Alka has the same dose of anti-inflammatory pain reliever as contained in Butazolidin. Butazolidin Alka, in addition, contains antacids.

When Prescribed: See Butazolidin.

Precautions and Warnings: See Butazolidin.

Side Effects and Adverse Reactions: See Butazolidin.

Butazolidin (Continued)

kidney stones, painful urination, high blood pressure, pain in the eyes, blurred vision, loss of hearing, increase in size of thyroid (in neck), general agitation, confusion, lethargy, salivary gland enlargement, headache, drowsiness, tremors, numbness, weakness, ringing in ears.

BUTISOL SODIUM® (McNeil Laboratories, Inc.)

Generic Name: Sodium butabarbital

Dosage Form	Strength	Route
Tablet	15 mg	Oral
	30 mg*	Oral
	50 mg	Oral
	100 mg	Oral
Capsule	15 mg	Oral
	30 mg	Oral
	50 mg	Oral
	100 mg	Oral
Elixir	30 mg/5 cc	Oral

When Prescribed: Butisol Sodium is a barbiturate prescribed as a sedative or a sleeping pill in patients where weaker medications are not deemed effective.

Precautions and Warnings: This drug should not be taken with other sedatives or sleeping pills, nor with alcohol or relaxants. Patients using this drug should not drive or operate machinery. Patients using any type of barbiturates for prolonged periods should seek the help of a physician when attempting to discontinue use. Abrupt cessation may be hazardous.

Side Effects and Adverse Reactions: Butisol Sodium may be habit forming. Individuals may develop a psychological dependence on this drug. People who have overused this drug may develop a physical dependence that will result in withdrawal symptoms including convulsions. Adverse reactions include hangover, drowsiness, lethargy, headache, skin eruptions, nausea, vomiting, hives.

CARBRITAL® KAPSEALS® (Parke, Davis and Company)

Generic Name: Pentobarbital sodium, carbromal

Dosage Form	Strength	Route
Capsule	Available in one	Oral
	strength only	Oral

When Prescribed: Carbrital, a barbiturate, contains a sleep-inducing agent and a sedative. The sleep-inducing agent acts rapidly, while the sedative continues its action. Carbrital is usually prescribed as a sleep-inducing drug in patients where less potent drugs are not effective.

Side Effects and Adverse Reactions: Carbrital sodium is a barbiturate which may be habit forming. Individuals may develop a psychological as well as physiological dependence on this drug. People who have overused this drug may develop a physical dependence that will result in withdrawal symptoms including convulsions. Patients using any type of barbiturates for prolonged periods should seek the help of a physician when attempting to discontinue use. Abrupt cessation may be hazardous. Adverse reactions include hangover, drowsiness, lethargy, headache, skin eruptions, nausea, vomiting, hives, loss of balance, pain, excitement, diarrhea.

CATAPRES® (Boehringer Ingelheim)

Generic Name: Clonidine hydrochloride

Dosage Form	Strength	Route
Tablet	0.1 mg	Oral
	0.2 mg	Oral

When Prescribed: Catapres is prescribed for the treatment of high blood pressure. Catapres is mild to moderate in potency and is often prescribed with other drugs to reduce high blood pressure.

Precautions and Warnings: If drowsiness occurs you should not drive or operate dangerous machinery. Catapres therapy should not be discontinued without consulting your physician. This drug may enhance the depressive effects of alcohol, sleeping pills, tranquilizers, and sedatives.

Side Effects and Adverse Reactions: Dry mouth, drowsiness, sedation, constipation, dizziness, headache, fatigue, loss of appetite, depression, nausea, vomiting, weight gain, enlargement of breasts, pains in hands or feet, nightmares, insomnia, nervousness, restlessness, anxiety, rash, hives, itching, thinning of hair, impotence, difficulties in urination, dryness of eyes or nose.

CHLORAL HYDRATE
The generic name for a drug produced by numerous companies in various forms and strengths. Also marketed as:
FELSULES® CAPSULES, Fellows;
KESSODRATE® CAPSULES, McKesson;
NOCTEC® CAPSULES, E. R. Squibb;
SK-CHLORAL HYDRATE, Smith Kline and French

Generic Name: Chloral hydrate

Dosage Form	Strength	Route
Capsule	500 mg	Oral

When Prescribed: Chloral hydrate is prescribed to induce sleep. Because it is not a barbiturate it is especially well suited for the ill, the young and the elderly.

Precautions and Warnings: Should not be taken in combination with alcohol, sedatives, relaxants or other sleeping pills. Patients should not drive or operate machinery after taking this drug. Should not be used longer than 2–3 weeks. Chloral hydrate may be habit forming, producing a psychological and physiological dependence.

Side Effects and Adverse Reactions: Stomach irritation, excitement, delirium.

CHLOR-TRIMETON® (Schering Corporation)

Generic Name: Chlorpheniramine maleate

Dosage Form	Strength	Route
Tablet	4 mg	Oral
Syrup	2 mg/5 cc	Oral
Time Release Tab	8 mg	Oral
	12 mg	Oral

When Prescribed: Chlor-Trimeton is an antihistamine prescribed for hay fever, allergic congestion, conjunctivitis (pinkeye) due to allergy, mild forms of hives and swelling due to allergy, prevention of skin reactions due to transfusions of blood or plasma, hypersensitivity of skin due to allergy, follow-up therapy for allergic reactions to drugs.

Precautions and Warnings: Since drowsiness may occur, Chlor-Trimeton should not be taken before undertaking any activity requiring full mental alertness such as driving or operating machinery. This drug should not be taken by nursing mothers. The safe use of Chlor-Trimeton in pregnancy has not been established.

Side Effects and Adverse Reactions: Drowsiness, restlessness, dry mouth, dizziness, weakness, loss of appetite, nausea, headache, nervousness, frequent urination, heartburn, double vision, painful urination, skin inflammation, rash, excessive perspiration, chills, dryness of mouth and nose and throat, sensitivity to sunlight, heart flutters, dizziness, confusion, restless-

CHOLEDYL (Parke-Davis)

Generic Name: Oxtriphylline

Dosage Form	Strength	Route
Tablet	200 mg	Oral
	100 mg	Oral
Elixir (contains alcohol)	100 mg/5 ml	Oral
Pediatric syrup	50 mg/5 ml	Oral

When Prescribed: Choledyl is prescribed to aid breathing in patients with asthma, bronchitis, or emphysema.

Precautions and Warnings: Use of this drug with other similar type drugs can produce adverse reactions, especially in children.

Side Effects and Adverse Reactions: Gastric distress, irregular heartbeat, nervous system stimulation.

CHLOR-TRIMETON (continued)

ness, tremors, loss of balance, ringing in ears, diarrhea, constipation, changes in menstrual pattern, thickening of bronchial secretions, tightness of chest, wheezing, nasal stuffiness.

Note: The 4 mg tablet, the 8 mg tablet, and the syrup can now be purchased without a prescription.

CLEOCIN® HCL CAPSULES (The Upjohn Company)

Generic Name: Clindamycin HCl hydrate

Dosage Form	Strength	Route
Capsule	75 mg	Oral
	150 mg	Oral

When Prescribed: Cleocin is prescribed for treatment of bacterial infections by susceptible organisms including those of the upper respiratory tract (nose, throat), lower respiratory tract (lungs, bronchial tubes), skin and gums.

Precautions and Warnings: Severe abdominal reactions can occur from the use of Cleocin. If any of the side effects or adverse reactions listed below occurs, Cleocin should be discontinued and your physician consulted. Safety for use in pregnancy has not been established.

Side Effects and Adverse Reactions: Abdominal pain, nausea, vomiting, severe diarrhea, rash, hives, fainting, yellowing of skin or eyes, super-infection by nonsusceptible organisms, pain in joints.

CLINORIL (Merck, Sharp and Dohme)

Generic Name: Sulindac

Dosage Form	Strength	Route
Tablet	150 mg	Oral
	200 mg	Oral

When Prescribed: Clinoril is prescribed for the relief of pain and inflammation from arthritis, bursitis, and other painful disorders of the joints.

Precautions and Warnings: This drug should not be taken by pregnant women or nursing mothers. It is not recommended that Clinoril and aspirin be taken together.

Side Effects and Adverse Reactions: Gastrointestinal pain, indigestion, nausea, vomiting, diarrhea, constipation, gas, loss of appetite, gastrointestinal cramps, rash, itching, dizziness, headache, nervousness, ringing in the ears, swelling, dryness of nose or throat, loss of balance, fever, skin rash, chills.

COGENTIN (Merck, Sharp and Dohme)

Generic Name: Benztropine mesylate

Dosage Form	Strength	Route
Tablet	0.5 mg	Oral
	1.0 mg	Oral
	2.0 mg	Oral

When Prescribed: Cogentin is prescribed to control the abnormal movements and muscle stiffness associated with Parkinson's disease and certain other diseases.

Precautions and Warnings: The safe use of this drug in pregnancy has not been established. Cogentin may impair the mental and/or physical abilities required to drive a car or operate dangerous machinery. Report any gastrointestinal upsets to your physician immediately. This drug may impair your ability to perspire. This could lead to a dangerous elevation in body temperature in hot environments.

Side Effects and Adverse Reactions: Dry mouth, blurred vision, nausea, nervousness, vomiting, constipation, numbness of the fingers, listlessness, depression, skin rash.

COLY-MYCIN ® S OTIC (Parke-Davis)

Generic Name: Colistin sulfate, neomycin sulfate, thonzonium bromide, hydrocortisone acetate otic suspension

Dosage Form	Strength	Route
Liquid	Available in one strength only	Otic (ear) drops

When Prescribed: Coly-mycin S Otic eardrops are prescribed for the treatment of bacterial infections of the external ear canal. They may also be prescribed for infections resulting from operations involving the ear.

Precautions and Warnings: Should not be warmed above body temperature in order to insure full potency.

Side Effects and Adverse Reactions: Sensitization or irritation of skin, super-infection by nonsusceptible organisms.

COMBID® SPANSULES®
(Smith Kline and French Laboratories)

Generic Name: Prochlorperazine maleate, isopropamide iodide

Dosage Form	Strength	Route
Capsule (Time Release)	Available in one strength only	Oral

When Prescribed: Combid is prescribed as therapy for peptic ulcer and various other gastrointestinal disorders. It is intended to reduce the amount of stomach secretion, reduce spasms and movements of the gastrointestinal tract, relieve anxiety and tension and control nausea and vomiting.

Precautions and Warnings: Should not be taken with sleeping pills, sedatives, alcohol or tranquilizers. If drowsiness occurs, patients should not operate motor vehicles or machinery.

Side Effects and Adverse Reactions: Dry mouth, urinary hesitancy and retention, increased heart rate, irregular heart beat, dilation of the pupils, inability of the eyes to accommodate to light changes, blurred vision, constipation, bloated feeling, difficulty swallowing, fever, nasal congestion, spasms or jerky movements, tremors, involuntary movements of the face, tongue, or jaws, drowsiness, dizziness, convulsions, headache, impotence, altered personality, low blood pressure, fainting, cardiac arrest, anemia and other blood disorders, yellowing of the skin, lactation, development of breasts in males, menstrual irregularities, false positive pregnancy tests, increased sensitivity to sunlight, itching, hives, rash allergic reactions, swelling, eye disorders.

COMPAZINE® (Smith Kline and French Laboratories)

Generic Name: Prochlorperazine maleate

Dosage Form	Strength	Route
Suppository	2.5 mg	Rectal
	5 mg*	Rectal
	25 mg	Rectal
Tablet	5 mg	Oral
	10 mg	Oral
	25 mg	Oral
Capsule	10 mg	Oral
(Time Release)	15 mg	Oral
(Spansules®)	30 mg	Oral
	75 mg	Oral
Syrup	5 mg/5ml	Oral

When Prescribed: Compazine is prescribed for certain psychotic disorders, for moderate to severe anxiety, and for control of severe nausea and vomiting.

Precautions and Warnings: Patients using Compazine may have impaired mental and/or physical abilities, especially during the first few days of therapy. Therefore, patients should not undertake potentially dangerous tasks such as driving or operating machinery. Compazine should not be taken with alcohol, tranquilizers, sedatives or sleeping pills. Compazine is a potent drug which must be used with caution. Patients noticing any unusual symptoms, including those listed below, should consult a physician immediately.

Side Effects and Adverse Reactions: Drowsiness, dizziness, absence of menstruation, skin disorders, low blood pressure, fainting, jerky movements, tremors, agitation, jitteriness, insomnia, muscle spasms, difficulty swallowing, spasms of eye muscles or tongue, difficulty walking, drooling,

CORDRAN® (Dista Products Company)

Generic Name: Flurandrenolide

Dosage Form	Strength	Route
Cream	.05% .025%	Topical (apply directly to affected area)
Lotion	.05%	
Ointment	.05% .025%	

When Prescribed: Cordran is a synthetic equivalent of a substance produced in the body. It is a potent agent prescribed to reduce itching, swelling and inflammation in certain skin disorders.

Precautions and Warnings: Cordran should not be used extensively, in large amounts over large areas, or for prolonged periods of time on pregnant patients.

Side Effects and Adverse Reactions: Skin eruptions, burning, dryness, irritated hair follicles, excessive hair growth, loss of pigment, irritation, itching, destruction of skin.

CORTISPORIN® OTIC DROPS
(Burroughs Wellcome Company)

Generic Name: Polymycin B sulfate, neomycin sulfate, hydrocortisone

Dosage Form	Strength	Route
Liquid	Available in one strength only	Otic (ear) drops

When Prescribed: Cortisporin Otic eardrops are prescribed for the treatment of bacterial infections of the external ear canal. They may also be prescribed for infections resulting from operations involving the ear.

Precautions and Warnings: To insure full potency, drops should not be warmed above body temperature. Shake well before using.

Side Effects and Adverse Reactions: Sensitization or irritation of skin, super-infection by nonsusceptible organisms.

Compazine (Continued)

abnormal uncontrolled facial movements, convulsions, headache, dryness of mouth, nasal congestion, nausea, constipation, intestinal blockage, impotence, cardiac arrest, anemia and other blood disorders, yellowing of skin, lactation, development of breasts in males, false positive pregnancy tests, increased sensitivity to sunlight, itching, hives, rash, allergic reactions, swelling, eye disorders, blurred vision.

COUMADIN® (Endo Laboratories, Inc.)

Generic Name: Crystalline sodium warfarin

Dosage Form	Strength	Route
Tablet	2 mg	Oral
	2.5 mg	Oral
	5 mg*	Oral
	7.5 mg	Oral
	10 mg	Oral
	25 mg	Oral

When Prescribed: Coumadin is prescribed for the prevention of blood clots in the veins, certain heart conditions that may lead to clots and clots in the lungs. This drug may also be prescribed for patients who have suffered mild strokes. The aim of Coumadin therapy is to impede the clotting mechanism of the blood, while avoiding spontaneous bleeding.

Precautions and Warnings: Should be taken under strict supervision where the clotting time of the blood is determined periodically. Should not be taken if any of the symptoms listed below appear. Coumadin taken with other drugs can lead to serious interactions. Notify your physician of all prescription and non-prescription drugs which you use. Should not be taken during pregnancy or by nursing mothers.

Side Effects and Adverse Reactions: Major or minor bleeding from any tissue or organ, loss of hair, hives, skin infections, fever, nausea, diarrhea, skin damage due to reduced blood supply, abdominal cramping.

CYCLOSPASMOL® (Ives Laboratories, Inc.)

Generic Name: Cyclandelate

Dosage Form	Strength	Route
Capsule	200 mg*	Oral
	400 mg	Oral
Tablet	100 mg	Oral

When Prescribed: Cyclospasmol is a drug which dilates (increases the diameter) of blood vessels so as to allow more blood to flow to areas that might otherwise be deprived of sufficient blood. It is used, along with other types of therapy, in leg cramps and limping caused by poor circulation; in cases where arteries have become clogged or blocked; in cases of blood clots; in cases of poor circulation to the hands and/or feet; and in cases of blood vessel disease in the brain.

Precautions and Warnings: Your physician should be notified if any of the symptoms listed below appears. The safe use of Cyclospasmol during pregnancy has not been established.

Side Effects and Adverse Reactions: Gastrointestinal distress, flushing, headache, weakness, rapid heartbeat.

DALMANE® (Roche Laboratories)

Generic Name: Flurazepam hydrochloride

Dosage Form	Strength	Route
Dosage Form	Strength	Route
Capsule	15 mg	Oral
	30 mg*	Oral

When Prescribed: Dalmane is a sleep-inducing agent useful in all types of insomnia characterized by difficulty in falling asleep, frequent nocturnal awakenings and/or early morning awakening.

Precautions and Warnings: This drug is not recommended for use in persons under 15 years of age. Patients should not combine Dalmane with alcohol, tranquilizers, sedatives or other sleeping pills. Patients should not drive or operate heavy machinery after taking this drug. The use of Dalmane during pregnancy should almost always be avoided.

Side Effects and Adverse Reactions: Dizziness, drowsiness, light-headedness, staggering, loss of balance, falling, severe sedation, lethargy, disorientation, coma, headache, heartburn, upset stomach, nausea, vomiting, diarrhea, constipation, gastrointestinal pain, nervousness, talkativeness, apprehension, irritability, weakness, fluttering of the heart, chest pains, body and joint pains, urinary-genital complaints, sweating, flushing, blurred vision, burning eyes, fainting, low blood pressure, shortness of breath, itching, skin rash, dry mouth, bitter taste, excessive salivation, loss of appetite, euphoria, depression, slurred speech, confusion, restlessness, hallucinations, excitement, stimulation, hyperactivity.

DARVOCET–N® (Eli Lilly and Co.)

Generic Name: Propoxyphene napsylate with acetaminophen

Dosage Form	Strength	Route
Tablet	50	Oral
	100*	Oral

When Prescribed: Darvocet–N is prescribed for the relief of mild to moderate pain, either when pain is present alone or when it is accompanied by fever. Darvocet–N contains a non-aspirin pain reliever and fever reducer that is well tolerated by people who are sensitive to aspirin.

Precautions and Warnings: Darvocet–N can cause a psychological and/or physical dependence and withdrawal symptoms. This preparation should not be ingested before undertaking potentially dangerous tasks such as driving or operating machinery, nor should it be taken with alcohol, sedatives, tranquilizers or sleeping pills. The safe use of this drug during pregnancy has not been established.

Side Effects and Adverse Reactions: Dizziness, drowsiness, nausea, vomiting, constipation, abdominal pains, skin rashes, lightheadedness, headache, weakness, euphoria, uneasiness and minor visual disturbances.

DARVON® (Eli Lilly and Company)

Generic Name: Propoxyphene hydrochloride

Dosage Form	Strength	Route
Capsule	32 mg	Oral
	65 mg*	Oral

When Prescribed: Darvon is prescribed for the relief of mild to moderate pain of any nature. If pain can be controlled with Darvon, it is preferred over stronger narcotic drugs.

Precautions and Warnings: Darvon has potential for abuse and dependency. This drug should not be taken with alcohol, tranquilizers, sedatives, sleeping pills, or other central-nervous system depressants. The safe use of this drug during pregnancy has not been established. Darvon is not recommended for children. If drowsiness occurs you should not drive or operate dangerous machinery.

Side Effects and Adverse Reactions: Dizziness, sedation, nausea, vomiting, constipation, abdominal pain, skin rashes, lightheadedness, headache, weakness, euphoria, uneasiness, minor visual disturbances.

DARVON® COMPOUND (Eli Lilly and Company)

Generic Name: Propoxyphene hydrochloride plus aspirin, phenacetin and caffeine

Dosage Form	Strength	Route
Capsule	32 mg	Oral
	65 mg*	Oral

When Prescribed: Darvon Compound is prescribed for the relief of mild to moderate pain of any nature. If pain can be controlled with Darvon, it is preferred over stronger narcotic drugs.

Precautions and Warnings: Darvon Compound should not be taken before undertaking potentially dangerous tasks such as driving or operating machinery. Should not be taken with alcohol, sedatives, tranquilizers or sleeping pills. Darvon Compound can produce drug dependence characterized by psychological dependence and, less frequently, physical dependence. The safe use of this drug in pregnancy has not been established. Darvon Compound is not recommended for children.

Side Effects and Adverse Reactions: Dizziness, tiredness, nausea and vomiting. Other adverse reactions include constipation, abdominal pain, skin rash, lightheadedness, headache, weakness, euphoria, uneasiness and minor visual disturbances.

DARVON–N® (Eli Lilly and Company)

Generic Name: Propoxyphene napsylate

Dosage Form	Strength	Route
Tablet	100 mg	Oral
Liquid	100 mg/10 ml	Oral

Note: Darvon–N in activity is identical to Darvon. The drugs differ in that Darvon–N can be made into tablets or a liquid. 100 mg of Darvon–N is required to deliver the same amount of pain reliever as 65 mg of Darvon.

Precautions and Warnings: See Darvon.

Side Effects and Adverse Reactions: See Darvon.

DECADRON® (Merck Sharp and Dohme)

Generic Name: Dexamethasone

Dosage Form	Strength	Route
Tablet	.25 mg	Oral
	.50 mg	Oral
	.75 mg*	Oral
	1.5 mg	Oral
	4.0 mg	Oral

When Prescribed: Decadron is the man-made equivalent of a substance which is produced naturally in your body by the adrenal glands. The main action of decadron is to reduce inflammation and swelling. Decadron is prescribed for a variety of reasons including glandular disorders, rheumatic and arthritic disorders, diseases of connective tissues, skin diseases, allergies, eye disorders, respiratory diseases, blood disorders, swelling, meningitis, tuberculosis, gastrointestinal diseases, swelling from dental work.

Precaution and Warnings: Mothers taking decadron should not nurse. Patients on Decadron therapy should not receive smallpox or other vaccinations. Prolonged use of Decadron may cause psychological and/or physical dependence and subsequent withdrawal symptoms.

Side Effects and Adverse Reactions: Fluid retention, swelling, muscle weakness, ulcer, stomach irritation, slow wound healing, increased sweating, allergic skin reactions, convulsions, dizziness, headache, menstrual irregularities, suppression of growth in children, bulging of the eyes, weight gain, increased appetite, nausea, depressed or "blue" feeling.

DECLOMYCIN® (Lederle Laboratories)

Generic Name: Demeclocycline hydrochloride

Dosage Form	Strength	Route
Capsule	150 mg	Oral
Tablet	75 mg	Oral
	150 mg	Oral
	300 mg	Oral
Syrup	75 mg/5 cc	Oral
Pediatric drops	60 mg/ml	Oral

When Prescribed: Declomycin is an effective antibiotic prescribed for many different types of infection. It is often used in place of penicillin in patients who are allergic to penicillin.

Precautions and Warnings: Declomycin should not be taken by persons overly sensitive to demeclocycline (tetracycline). This drug should not be taken by children under eight or pregnant women. Do not use concomitantly with antacids containing magnesium, calcium or aluminum.

Side Effects and Adverse Reactions: Photosensitivity can occur while taking this drug. The following adverse reactions have been reported: superinfection by nonsusceptible organisms, loss of appetite, nausea, vomiting, diarrhea, inflammation of the tongue, difficulty in swallowing, stomachache, inflammation of the bowel and genital regions, skin rash, hives, swelling, shock.

DEMEROL.® (Winthrop Laboratories)

Generic Name: Meperidene hydrochloride

Dosage Form	Strength	Route
Tablet	50 mg*	Oral
	100 mg	Oral
Liquid	50 mg/5 cc	Oral

When Prescribed: Demerol is prescribed for the relief of moderate to severe pain of all types when non-narcotic pain relievers are not deemed effective.

Precautions and Warnings: Demerol should not be taken before undertaking any potentially hazardous task such as driving or operating machinery. Should not be taken with tranquilizers, pain relievers, sedatives, alcohol or sleeping pills.

Side Effects and Adverse Reactions: Demerol is a narcotic which may be habit forming. Lightheadedness, dizziness, nausea, vomiting and sweating, euphoria, uneasiness, weakness, headache, tremor, uncoordinated muscle movements, hallucinations, disorientation, visual disturbances, dry mouth, constipation, upset stomach, flushing of face, irregular heart beat, fainting, inability to urinate, itching, hives, skin rash.

DEMULEN® (Searle and Company)

Generic Name: Ethynodiol diacetate with ethinyl estradrol

Dosage Form	Strength	Route
Tablet	Available in one strength only	Oral

When Prescribed: Demulen is an oral contraceptive combining estrogen and progesterone.

Precautions and Warnings: An increased risk of blood clots and other serious disorders have been associated with the use of hormonal contraceptives such as Demulen. Oral contraceptives should be taken only under supervision of a physician. A booklet has been prepared to provide you with additional information. Ask your physician for this booklet. If any of the symptoms listed below appear, discuss continued use of the drug with a physician. Cigarette smoking increases the risk of heart and circulatory trouble as side effects of oral contraceptive use. Women who use oral contraceptives should not smoke.

Side Effects and Adverse Reactions: Nausea, vomiting, stomach cramps, bleeding or spotting at times other than during "period," changes in amount of menstrual flow, absence of menstruation, swelling, abnormal darkening of skin, changes in breasts including tenderness, enlargement, secretion, an increase or decrease in weight, suppression of lactation when taken immediately after childbirth, migraine, rash, rise in blood pressure, mental depression, changes in sex drive, changes in appetite, headache, nervousness, dizziness, fatigue, backache, increase in facial hair, loss of scalp hair, itching.

DIABINESE® (Pfizer Laboratories Division)

Generic Name: Chlorpropamide

Dosage Form	Strength	Route
Tablet	100 mg	Oral
	250 mg*	Oral

When Prescribed: Diabinese is an oral substance that will reduce sugar levels in the blood of adult patients with mild or moderately severe diabetes (diabetes mellitus) which cannot be controlled by diet alone. It can often replace the need for insulin in these patients and is frequently prescribed in conjunction with other oral blood sugar-reducing agents. It is generally not prescribed for children with diabetes.

Precautions and Warnings: The use of alcohol, sedatives, sleeping pills, certain pain relievers or tranquilizers with Diabinese may lead to adverse side effects. Your physician should be consulted immediately if any side effect or adverse reaction occurs.

Side Effects and Adverse Reactions: Hives, rash, itching, water retention, yellowing of skin or eyes, dark urine, light-colored stools, low-grade fever, sore throat, diarrhea, anemia, loss of appetite, nausea, vomiting, heartburn, weakness, numbness, increased sensitivity to sunlight. If alcohol is taken during the Diabinese treatment, unusual flushing of skin on the face and neck may occur.

43

DIAMOX® (Lederle Laboratories)

Generic Name: Acetazolamide

Dosage Form	Strength	Route
Tablet	125 mg	Oral
	250 mg	Oral
Capsule	500 mg	Oral

When Prescribed: Diamox is prescribed for edema (water accumulation), epilepsy, and glaucoma. This drug is an enzyme inhibitor effective in the control of fluid secretion.

Precautions and Warnings: Diamox is not recommended for use during pregnancy.

Side Effects and Adverse Reactions: Fever, rash, kidney stones, abnormal skin sensations, loss of appetite, frequent urination, drowsiness, confusion, rash, paralysis, convulsions.

DIGOXIN The generic name for a drug produced by numerous companies in various forms and strengths.

Generic Name: Digoxin

Dosage Form	Strength	Route
Tablet	0.25 mg*	Oral

When Prescribed: Digoxin is a drug which increases the strength of the contractions of the heart. It is prescribed for patients with various forms of heart disease. It may also be used to control an irregular heart beat.

Precautions and Warnings: Digoxin is a potent drug which can cause serious side effects, particularly if taken in excess. Digoxin should be taken only under the close supervision of a physician to whom any side effects or adverse reactions should be reported.

Side Effects and Adverse Reactions: Loss of appetite, excessive salivation, nausea, vomiting, diarrhea, lethargy, drowsiness, confusion, visual disturbances, blurred vision, changes in color perception, irregular heart beat, headache, weakness, apathy.

DILANTIN® KAPSEALS® (Parke, Davis and Company)

Generic Name: Diphenylhydantoin sodium

Dosage Form	Strength	Route
Capsule (Kapseals®)	30 mg	Oral
	100 mg*	Oral
Liquid	30 mg/5 ml	Oral
	125 mg/5 ml	Oral
Kapseals® D.A.	100 mg	Oral
Tablet (Infatabs)	50 mg	Oral

When Prescribed: Dilantin Kapseals is prescribed for the control of convulsions in patients with epilepsy or in patients with other types of seizures. It may also be used to control an irregular heart beat.

Precautions and Warnings: Gum disorders occur frequently when this drug is used. The incidence of such disorders may be reduced by good oral hygiene including gum massage, frequent brushing and appropriate dental care. Should be taken with meals to help prevent gastric irritation.

Side Effects and Adverse Reactions: Abnormal eye movements, loss of balance, slurred speech, confusion, dizziness, insomnia, nervousness, twitching, headache, nausea, vomiting, constipation, fever, rash, anemia, enlargement of lymph glands, diseases of the joints, beard growth, hepatitis.

DIMETANE® (A. H. Robins Company)

Generic Name: Brompheniramine Maleate

Dosage Form	Strength	Route
Tablet (Time Release)	4 mg	Oral
Extentab (Time Release)	8 mg	Oral
Extentab	12 mg	Oral
Elixir	2 mg/5 ml	Oral

When Prescribed: Dimetane is an antihistamine which may be prescribed for relief of symptoms resulting from allergies, sinus infection, hay fever, conjunctivitis (pink eye), swollen eyes, allergies from blood transfusions, skin allergies.

Precautions and Warnings: Dimetane is not recommended for use during pregnancy. This drug should not be taken with alcohol, sleeping pills, sedatives, or tranquilizers. If drowsiness should occur do not drive or operate dangerous machinery.

Side Effects and Adverse Reactions: Rash, itching, sensitivity to sunlight, excessive perspiration, chills, dryness of mouth, nose, throat, headache, irregular heart beat, dizziness, loss of coordination, confusion, restlessness, excitation, nervousness, tremors, irritability, euphoria, numbness or tingling of skin, blurred vision, double vision, loss of balance, ringing in ears, hysteria, convulsions, loss of appetite, nausea, vomiting, diarrhea, constipation, urinary difficulties, menstrual irregularities, thickening of bronchial secretions, tightness in chest, wheezing, nasal stuffiness, changes in personality such as irritability, nervousness.

45

DIMETANE® EXPECTORANT
DIMETANE® EXPECTORANT–DC
(A. H. Robins Company)

Generic Name: Brompheniramine maleate, guaifenesin, phenylephrine hydrochloride, phenylpropanolamine hydrochloride, alcohol, codeine phosphate (found in Dimetane Expectorant–DC only)

Dosage Form	Strength	Route
Liquid	Available in one strength only	Oral

When Prescribed: Dimetane Expectorant is prescribed for the relief of cough and thinning of mucus, and for the relief of symptoms of allergy. Dimetane Expectorant–DC is prescribed for the same disorders when the additional cough-suppressive action of codeine is necessary.

Precautions and Warnings: Not recommended for use during pregnancy. Patients are cautioned against engaging in operations which require alertness. Dimetane Expectorant–DC contains codeine, which may be habit forming.

Side Effects and Adverse Reactions: Rash, hives, drowsiness, lassitude, nausea, dryness of the mouth, dilation of pupils, excitement, irritability, excessive perspiration, chills, headache, heart flutters, rapid heart beat, sedation, blurred vision, ringing in ears, double vision, convulsions, dizziness, confusion, fatigue, restlessness, excitation, nervousness, shaking, insomnia, euphoria, loss of appetite, vomiting, diarrhea, constipation, urinary problems, tightness of chest, wheezing, nasal stuffiness, tingling, heaviness, weakness of hands.

DIMETAPP® EXTENTABS®
(A. H. Robins Company)

Generic Name: Brompheniramine maleate, phenylephrine hydrochloride, phenylpropanolamine hydrochloride

Dosage Form	Strength	Route
Tablets (Time Release)	Available in one strength only	Oral
Elixir	120 ml	Oral

When Prescribed: Dimetapp is an antihistamine and decongestant prescribed for the relief of symptoms of allergies of the upper respiratory tract including the common cold, seasonal allergies, sinus infections, hay fever, conjunctivitis (pinkeye), swollen eyes.

Precautions and Warings: Should not be combined with alcohol, sleeping pills, sedatives or tranquilizers. Activities which require alertness, such as driving, should be avoided.

Side Effects and Adverse Reactions: Rash, hives, anemia, drowsiness, lassitude, giddiness, dryness of mucous membranes, tightness of the chest, thickening of bronchial secretions, painful and frequent urination, fluttering of the heart, changes in blood pressure, headache, fainting, dizziness, ringing in the ears, incoordination, visual disturbances, dilation of pupils, depression, stimulation, loss of appetite, nausea, vomiting, diarrhea, constipation, heartburn.

DIURIL® (Merck Sharp and Dohme)

Generic Name: Chlorothiazide MSD

Dosage Form	Strength	Route
Tablet	250 mg	Oral
	500 mg*	Oral
Liquid	250 mg/5 ml	Oral

When Prescribed: Diuril is prescribed as an agent which helps the body pass water and salt in patients who retain water due to a variety of reasons. It is also prescribed for the reduction of blood pressure in patients with high blood pressure.

Precautions and Warnings: Mothers should not nurse while taking this drug.

Side Effects and Adverse Reactions: Weakness, lethargy, drowsiness, restlessness, muscle pains or cramps, muscle fatigue, low blood pressure, frequent urination, rapid heartbeat, nausea, vomiting, loss of appetite, diarrhea, constipation, yellowing of skin or eyes, gastrointestinal distress, dizziness, numbness, headache, yellow appearance of objects, anemia, rash, hives, increased sensitivity to sunlight, fever, respiratory distress, blurred vision.

DONNAGEL®–PG (A. H. Robins Company)

Generic Name: Kaolin, hyoscyamine sulfate, atropine sulfate, hyoscine hydrobromide, alcohol, opium, pectin

Dosage Form	Strength	Route
Liquid	Available in one strength only	Oral

When Prescribed: Donnagel–PG is prescribed for the control of acute, nonspecific diarrhea where milder, nonprescription drugs are not considered effective.

Precautions and Warnings: Donnagel–PG contains opium, which may be habit forming.

Side Effects and Adverse Reactions: Blurring of vision, dry mouth, difficult urination, flushing and dryness of the skin, irregular heart beat, constipation.

DONNATAL® (A. H. Robins Company)

Generic Name: Hyoscyamine sulfate, atropine sulfate, hyoscine hydrobromide, phenobarbital, alcohol (liquid only)

Dosage Form	Strength	Route
Tablet	Each form is	Oral
Capsule	available in one	Oral
No. 2 Tablets	strength only	Oral
Liquid (Elixir)		Oral
Time Release Tablet		Oral

When Prescribed: Donnatal is prescribed for the treatment of ulcers and other forms of intestinal distress.

Precautions and Warnings: Donnatal contains phenabarbital, which may be habit forming.

Side Effects and Adverse Reactions: Blurred vision, dry mouth, difficult urination, flushing or dryness of the skin.

DORIDEN® (USV Development Corp.)

Generic Name: Glutethimide

Dosage Form	Strength	Route
Tablet	250 mg	Oral
	500 mg*	Oral
Capsule	500 mg	Oral

When Prescribed: Doriden is prescribed to induce sleep in people who have chronic difficulty falling asleep or who awaken frequently during the night.

Precautions and Warnings: Should not be taken with antidepressants, alcohol, tranquilizers or sedatives. Doriden acts rapidly. After taking this drug you should not engage in any activity requiring complete alertness. Although Doriden is not a narcotic, both physical and psychological dependence on this drug can occur with overuse. Doriden is not recommended for use during pregnancy or for use in children.

Side Effects and Adverse Reactions: Rash, hives, nausea, drug hangover, excitation, blurring of vision.

DRIXORAL® (Schering Corporation)

Generic Name: Dexbrompheniramine maleate, pseudoephedrine sulfate

Dosage Form	Strength	Route
Tablet	Available in one strength only	Oral

When Prescribed: Drixoral is an antihistamine prescribed for relief of symptoms of upper respiratory congestion in allergies and hay fever. It is also prescribed for relief of pressure in nasal sinuses, and eustachian tubes.

Precautions and Warnings: Drixoral is usually not prescribed for children under 12 nor for pregnant women or nursing mothers. This preparation should not be taken with alcohol, tranquilizers, sedatives, sleeping pills. Activities involving mental alertness should be avoided.

Side Effects and Adverse Reactions: Drowsiness, confusion, restlessness, nausea, vomiting, rash, loss of balance, irregular heart beat, loss of appetite, dizziness, painful urination, headache, insomnia, anxiety, tension, weakness, rapid heartbeat, sweating, blood pressure elevation, dilation of pupils, gastric distress, abdominal cramps, stimulation.

DYAZIDE® (Smith Kline and French Laboratories)

Generic Name: Triamterene, hydrochlorothiazide

Dosage Form	Strength	Route
Capsule	Available in one strength only	Oral

When Prescribed: Dyazide is prescribed to help pass water and salt in patients who retain abnormal amounts of water due to a variety of diseases. It is also prescribed for treatment of mild to moderate high blood pressure. Dyazide is prescribed only after your physician has determined that the fixed combination of drugs is correct for you.

Precautions and Warnings: Dyazide is a potent drug. Any abnormal effects should be reported immediately to your physician.

Side Effects and Adverse Reactions: Muscle cramps, weakness, dizziness, headache, dry mouth, fainting, rash, hives, increased sensitivity to sunlight, nausea, vomiting, diarrhea, constipation, numbness, yellow vision.

E.E.S.® (Abbott Laboratories)

Generic Name: Erythromycin®
ethylsuccinate

Dosage Form	Strength	Route
Chewable tablet	200 mg	Oral
Infants' drops	100 mg/dropper	Oral
Liquid	200 mg/ teaspoon	Oral
	400 mg/ teaspoon	Oral
Granules for suspension	200 mg/ teaspoon (5cc)	Oral
Tablet	400 mg	Oral

When Prescribed: E.E.S. is prescribed for a wide variety of infections. It is often prescribed for infections where penicillin would normally be the drug of choice but the patient has a sensitivity to penicillin.

Precautions and Warnings: E.E.S. is an antibiotic which can cause an allergic reaction. The safety of this drug during pregnancy has not been established.

Side Effects and Adverse Reactions: Abdominal cramping or discomfort, nausea, vomiting, diarrhea, super infection by nonsusceptible organisms, hives, rash, fainting.

ELAVIL® (Merck Sharp and Dohme)

Generic Name: Amitriptyline HCl

Dosage Form	Strength	Route
Tablet	10 mg*	Oral
	25 mg	Oral
	50 mg	Oral
	75 mg	Oral
	100 mg	Oral
	150 mg	Oral

When Prescribed: Elavil is prescribed for the relief of symptoms of mental depression or mental depression accompanied by anxiety.

Precautions and Warnings: This drug may impair mental and/or physical abilities required for performance of hazardous tasks such as operating machinery or driving a motor vehicle. It is not recommended for use by children under 12 years of age. Elavil may enhance the response to alcohol and other depressants such as tranquilizers, sleeping pills and sedatives. The safe use of Elavil in pregnancy has not been established.

Side Effects and Adverse Reactions: Decreases in blood pressure, rapid heart rate, irregular heart beat upon rising from lying or sitting, stroke, confusional states, disturbed concentration, disorientation, delusions, hallucinations, excitement, anxiety, restlessness, insomnia, nightmares, numbness, tingling, incoordination, loss of balance, tremors, seizures, ringing in the ears, dry mouth, blurred vision, discomfort of eyes, constipation, inability to urinate, rash, hives, increased sensitivity of skin to light, swelling of face and tongue, anemia, nausea, vomiting, heartburn, loss of appetite, peculiar

ELIXOPHYLLIN® (Berlex Laboratories Inc.)

Generic Name: Theophylline, alcohol

Dosage Form	Strength	Route
Liquid Elixir)	Available in one strength only	Oral
Capsule	100 mg	Oral
	200 mg	Oral
Time Release Capsule	125 mg	Oral
	250 mg	Oral

When Prescribed: Elixophyllin is prescribed for relief of symptoms from bronchial asthma, emphysema, and other lung diseases characterized by difficulty in breathing.

Precautions and Warnings: Elixophyllin may interact with other drugs. Notify your physician if you are taking any other medication.

Side Effects and Adverse Reactions: Elixophyllin is generally well tolerated when taken at prescribed dosage levels.

Elavil (Continued)

tastes, diarrhea, swollen glands, black tongue, swelling of testicles and enlargement of breasts in males, increased breast size and excessive milk flow in females, changes in sex drive, dizziness, weakness, fatigue, headache, considerable weight change, increased perspiration, frequent urination, dilation of pupils, drowsiness, yellowing of skin or eyes, loss of hair. Abrupt cessation after long-term therapy may cause headache, weakness and fatigue.

EMPIRIN with CODEINE (Burroughs Wellcome Company)

Generic Name: Aspirin, Codeine

Dosage Form	Strength	Route
Tablet	No. 2	Oral
	No. 3	Oral
	No. 4	Oral

When Prescribed: Empirin with codeine is prescribed for the relief of mild, moderate, and moderate to severe pain. No. 4 contains the most codeine and is prescribed for moderate to severe pain. Nos. 2 and 3 are prescribed for less severe pain.

Precautions and Warnings: This drug contains codeine which may be habit forming. Should be used with caution when taking nervous system depressants such as tranquilizers, sleeping pills, sedatives, or alcohol. If drowsiness occurs you should not drive or operate dangerous machinery.

Side Effects and Adverse Reactions: Light-headedness, dizziness, sedation, nausea, vomiting, mood changes, constipation, itching, headache, loss of balance, ringing in the ears, mental confusion, drowsiness, sweating, thirst, stomach upset, rash.

E–MYCIN® (The Upjohn Company)

Generic Name: Erythromycin

Dosage Form	Strength	Route
Tablet	250 mg	Oral

When Prescribed: E–Mycin is prescribed for a wide variety of infections. It is often prescribed for infections where penicillin would normally be the drug of choice but the patient has a sensitivity to pencillin.

Precautions and Warnings: E–Mycin is an antibiotic which can cause an allergic reaction in susceptible individuals. The safe use of this drug in pregnancy has not been established.

Side Effects and Adverse Reactions: The most frequent side effects of erythromycin preparations are gastrointestinal, such as abdominal cramping, discomfort, nausea, vomiting and diarrhea. Other reactions include super-infection by nonsusceptible organisms, hives, rash and fainting.

ENDURON® (Abbott Laboratories)

Generic Name: Methyclothiazide

Dosage Form	Strength	Route
Tablet	2.5 mg	Oral
	5 mg	Oral

When Prescribed: Enduron is prescribed for treatment of high blood pressure, fluid accumulation due to congestive heart failure, cirrhosis of the liver, kidney disease, and other conditions where water accumulation is a symptom. Enduron helps the kidneys to pass water and salt thereby reducing water retention.

Precautions and Warnings: Enduron is a potent drug that should be used only under close supervision of your physician. This drug should not be taken by nursing mothers.

Side Effects and Adverse Reactions: Dryness of mouth, thirst, weakness, lethargy, drowsiness, restlessness, muscle pains or cramps, muscular fatigue, frequent urination, rapid heart beat, nausea, vomiting, loss of appetite, gastric upset, gastrointestinal cramps, constipation, dizziness, loss of balance, abnormal skin sensation, headache, rash, hives, skin eruptions, jaundice, yellow appearance of objects, diarrhea, sensitivity to sunlight.

EQUAGESIC® (Wyeth Laboratories)

Generic Name: Meprobamate, ethoheptazine citrate, acetyl-salicylic acid

Dosage Form	Strength	Route
Tablet	Available in one strength only	Oral

When Prescribed: Equagesic is Equanil with aspirin and an additional pain reliever. It is prescribed for the same reasons as Equanil, but in cases where the patient is experiencing mild pain.

Precautions and Warnings: See Equanil.

Side Effects and Adverse Reactions: See Equanil.

EQUANIL® (Wyeth Laboratories)

Generic Name: Meprobamate

Dosage Form	Strength	Route
Tablet	200 mg	Oral
	400 mg*	Oral
Capsule	400 mg	Oral
Liquid	200 mg/5 ml	Oral

When Prescribed: Equanil is prescribed for the relief of anxiety and tension, often in patients with various disease states which lead to anxiety and tension. It is also used to promote sleep in tense, anxious patients.

Precautions and Warnings: Overuse of this drug can lead to physical and/or phsychological dependence. Sudden withdrawal after prolonged and excessive use may cause adverse reactions. Equanil may impair the mental or physical abilities required for the performance of potentially hazardous tasks such as driving or operating machinery. Should not be taken with alcohol, tranquilizers, sedatives or sleeping pills. Equanil is not recommended for pregnant women, nursing mothers or children under 6.

Side Effects and Adverse Reactions: Drowsiness, loss of balance, dizziness, slurred speech, headache, weakness, tingling, crawling skin, inability of eyes to adapt to changing light, euphoria, stimulation, excitement, nausea, vomiting, diarrhea, irregular heart beat, fainting, itching, rash, hives, anemia, swelling, fever, chills.

ERYTHROCIN® STEARATE
(Abbott Laboratories)

Generic Name: Erythromycin stearate

Dosage Form	Strength	Route
Tablet	125 mg	Oral
(Filmtab®)	250 mg*	Oral
	500 mg	Oral

When Prescribed: Erythrocin is prescribed for a wide variety of infections. It is often prescribed for infections where penicillin would normally be the drug of choice but the patient has a sensitivity to penicillin.

Precautions and Warnings: Erythrocin is an antibiotic which can cause an allergic reaction in susceptible individuals. Best absorption is on an empty stomach. The safe use of this drug during pregnancy has not been established.

Side Effects and Adverse Reactions: Abdominal cramping, discomfort, nausea, vomiting and diarrhea, super-infection by nonsusceptible organisms, hives, rash and fainting.

ERYTHROMYCIN
The generic name for a drug produced by numerous companies in various forms and strengths. Also marketed as:
ERYTHROCIN®, Abbott;
PEDIAMYCIN®, Ross;
E–MYCIN®, Upjohn;
PFIZER–E®, Pfizer.

Generic Name: Erythromycin

Dosage Form	Strength	Route
Tablet	250 mg*	Oral

When Prescribed: Erythromycin is prescribed for a wide variety of infections. It is often prescribed for infections where penicillin would normally be the drug of choice but the patient has a sensitivity to penicillin.

Precautions and Warnings: Erythromycin is an antibiotic which can cause an allergic reaction in susceptible individuals. The safe use of this drug in pregnancy has not been established.

Side Effects and Adverse Reactions: The most frequent side effects of erythromycin preparations are gastrointestinal, such as abdominal cramping, discomfort, nausea, vomiting and diarrhea. Other reactions include super-infection by nonsusceptible organisms, hives, rash and fainting.

ESIDRIX® (Ciba Pharmaceutical Company)

Generic Name: Hydrochlorothiazide

Dosage Form	Strength	Route
Tablet	25 mg	Oral
	50 mg*	Oral
	100 mg	Oral

When Prescribed: Esidrix is a drug used to treat high blood pressure. It is also used to treat water retention due to various disorders. Esidrix is a diuretic, which helps rid the body of water and salt.

Precautions and Warnings: This drug is not for simple water retention due to pregnancy. Esidrix should not be taken by nursing mothers. Drugs such as Esidrix can disturb water and salt balance leading to serious complications. If you notice any of the side effects or adverse reactions listed below, consult your physician immediately.

Side Effects and Adverse Reactions: Dryness of mouth, thirst, weakness, "run down" feeling, drowsiness, restlessness, muscle pains or cramps, muscular fatigue, rapid heart beat, loss of appetite, stomach irritation, nausea, vomiting, intestinal cramps, diarrhea, constipation, dizziness, loss of balance, tingling of skin, headache, yellow appearance of objects, fainting, rash.

Etrafon (Continued)

tingling in the extremities, swelling of testicles, development of breasts in males, abnormal secretion from breasts in females, change in sex drive, chest pains, increased perspiration, loss of hair, abnormal change in weight.

ETRAFON® (Schering Corporation)

Generic Name: Perphenazine
NF — amitriptyline hydrochloride

Dosage Form	Strength	Route
Tablet	2–10	Oral
	4–10	Oral
	2–25	Oral
(Etrafon/forte)	4–25	Oral

When Prescribed: Etrafon is prescribed for certain psychological conditions in which moderate to severe anxiety, agitation and depression may be symptoms.

Precautions and Warnings: Etrafon is a potent drug that can have serious interactions with other drugs you may be taking; therefore inform your physician of all drugs you take. This drug should not be taken with alcohol, tranquilizers, sedatives or sleeping pills unless directed. Patients taking Etrafon should not drive or operate dangerous machinery. The safe use of this drug during pregnancy or by nursing mothers has not been established. Etrafon is not recommended for use in children.

Side Effects and Adverse Reactions: Uncontrolled movements of face or extremities, loss of balance, severe dizziness, shaking, increased sensitivity to sunlight, itching, rash, skin eruptions, asthma, dry mouth, salivation, headache, nausea, vomiting, loss of appetite, constipation, urinary difficulties, blurred vision, nasal congestion, excitement, lactation, changes in menstrual cycle, muscle weakness, lassitude, insomnia, swelling of face and tongue, visual difficulty, heart flutters, confusion, disorientation, numbness or

FASTIN (Beecham Laboratories)

Generic Name: Phentermine hydrochloride

Dosage Form	Strength	Route
Capsule	Available in one strength only	Oral

When Prescribed: Fastin is prescribed for a short period of time (usually a few weeks) in conjunction with a diet for the reduction of body weight in people who are overweight and cannot lose weight by diet alone.

Precautions and Warnings: Fastin may interfere with your ability to drive or operate machinery. This drug is related to the class of compounds known as amphetamines and, therefore, has potential for abuse and drug dependency. Fastin should not be used by children under 12.

Side Effects and Adverse Reactions: Heart flutters, excessive stimulation, restlessness, dizziness, insomnia, mood changes, tremor, headache, psychotic behavior, dryness of mouth, unpleasant taste, diarrhea, constipation, rash, changes in sex drive, impotence.

FEOSOL® (Menley and James Laboratories)

Generic Name: Ferrous sulfate (alcohol in elixir)

Dosage Form	Strength	Route
Liquid (elixir)	Available in one strength only	Oral
Timed Release spansule®	Available in one strength only	Oral
Tablet	Available in one strength only	Oral

When Prescribed: Feosol contains an essential mineral, iron. It is prescribed for use in cases of iron deficiency as in iron deficiency anemia.

Precautions and Warnings: Feosol may interfere with oral tetracycline absorption. Feosol and tetracycline should not be ingested within two hours of each other.

Side Effects and Adverse Reactions: Nausea, constipation, diarrhea.

Note: This drug is available without a prescription.

FERROUS SULFATE: The generic name for a drug produced by numerous companies in various strengths and forms. Also marketed as:
FEOSOL, Menley and James Laboratories; FERO-GRADUMET, Abbott.

Generic Name: Ferrous sulfate

Dosage Form	Strength	Route
Available in different forms and strengths		

When Prescribed: Ferrous sulfate supplies an essential mineral, iron. It is prescribed for cases of iron deficiency such as iron deficiency anemia.

Precautions and Warnings: Ferrous sulfate may interfere with oral tetracycline absorption. Ferrous sulfate and tetracycline should not be taken within two hours of each other.

Side Effects and Adverse Reactions: Nausea, constipation, diarrhea.

Note: In some dosages ferrous sulfate can be purchased without a prescription.

FIORINAL® (Sandoz Pharmaceuticals)

Generic Name: Butalbital, caffeine, aspirin, phenacetin

Dosage Form	Strength	Route
Tablet	Available in one strength only	Oral
Capsule	Available in one strength only	Oral

When Prescribed: Fiorinal is a combination of a mild sedative and pain reducer. It is prescribed for relief of pain of nervous tension headache or any pain brought on by tension or anxiety. It is also prescribed for reduction of pain and/or fever in conditions such as arthritis, menstrual cramps, the common cold and dental extractions.

Precautions and Warnings: Fiorinal contains a barbiturate which may be habit forming. Excessive or prolonged use should be avoided. If drowsiness occurs you should not drive or operate dangerous machinery. Fiorinal should not be used in children under 12.

Side Effects and Adverse Reactions: Drowsiness, nausea, dizziness, rash, lightheadedness, flatulence.

FIORINAL® with CODEINE (Sandoz Pharmaceutical)

Generic Name: Butalbital, caffeine, aspirin, phenacetin, codeine phosphate

Dosage Form	Strength	Route
Capsule	7.5 mg	Oral
	15 mg	Oral
	30 mg	Oral

When Prescribed: Fiorinal with Codeine is prescribed for the relief of pain resulting from a variety of conditions. It may also reduce the urge to cough, making it useful for respiratory infections, acute colds, bronchitis, and other conditions in which cough and pain are symptoms.

Precautions and Warnings: Fiorinal may be habit forming. If drowsiness occurs you should not drive or operate dangerous machinery.

Side Effects and Adverse Reactions: Nausea, vomiting, constipation, dizziness, skin rash, drowsiness, change in pupil size.

FLAGYL® (Searle and Company)

Generic Name: Metronidazole

Dosage Form	Strength	Route
Tablet	250 mg*	Oral

When Prescribed: Flagyl is prescribed for treatment of certain infections (trichomoniasis) of the genital tract in both males and females. It is also prescribed for treatment of dysentery (amebic dysentery) and liver abscess caused by amebas.

Precautions and Warnings: Alcoholic beverages should not be consumed during Flagyl therapy because abdominal cramps, vomiting and flushing may occur. This drug is not recommended for use during early pregnancy. Should not be used by nursing mothers.

Side Effects and Adverse Reactions: Nausea, headache, loss of appetite, vomiting, diarrhea, heartburn, cramps, constipation, unpleasant metallic taste, furry tongue, sore throat, dizziness, incoordination, loss of balance, numbness, crawling skin, joint pains, confusion, irritability, depression, insomnia, rash, weakness, hives, dryness of mouth, itching, painful urination, fever, painful sexual intercourse, frequent urination, decreased sex drive, nasal congestion, pus in urine, inflammation of bowel, darkening of urine, super-infection by nonsusceptible organisms.

FLEXERIL (Merck Sharpe and Dohme)

Generic Name: Cyclobenzaprine

Dosage Form	Strength	Route
Tablet	10 mg	Oral

When Prescribed: Flexeril is prescribed along with rest and physical therapy for the relief of muscle spasms or stiffness associated with disorders of the muscles or skeleton. Flexeril is usually only to be taken for a period of two to three weeks.

Precautions and Warnings: Flexeril may impair your physical and/or mental ability to drive or operate machinery. This drug should not be taken by nursing mothers or by children under 15.

Side Effects and Adverse Reactions: Drowsiness, dry mouth, dizziness, increased heart rate, weakness, fatigue, indigestion, nausea, abnormal sensations in skin, unpleasant taste, blurred vision, insomnia, sweating, muscle pains, breathing difficulties, abdominal pain, constipation, coated tongue, tremors, joint pain, euphoria, nervousness, disorientation, confusion, headache, urinary difficulties, loss of coordination, mood depression, hallucinations, rash, swelling of face or tongue, heart flutters, disturbed concentration, delusions, excitement, anxiety, nightmares, seizures, ringing in the ears, eye problems, increased sensitivity to sunlight, vomiting, loss of appetite, upset stomach, swollen glands, black tongue, yellowing of skin, swelling of testicle and development of breasts in males, increase in breast size and secretion in females, changes in sex drive, weight gain or loss, loss of hair.

GANTANOL® (Roche Laboratories)

Generic Name: Sulfamethoxazole

Dosage Form	Strength	Route
Tablet	1 gm	Oral
	0.5 gm	Oral
Liquid	0.5 gm/5cc	Oral

When Prescribed: Gantanol is a sulfonamide, which is an antibacterial agent used to treat urinary tract infections, meningitis, ear infections and various other infections.

Precautions and Warnings: Gantanol is usually not prescribed during pregnancy at term or during the nursing period. Should be taken with adequate fluid intake.

Side Effects and Adverse Reactions: Sore throat, fever, paleness, yellowing of the skin or eyes, rash, anemia, generalized skin eruptions, hives, itching, swelling, fainting, eye infections, increased sensitivity to sunlight, nausea, vomiting, abdominal pains, hepatitis, diarrhea, loss of appetite, headache, pains in extremities, mental depression, loss of balance, ringing in the ear, dizziness, insomnia, fever, chills, frequent urination, lack of urination, super-infection by nonsusceptible organisms.

GANTRISIN® (Roche Laboratories)

Generic Name: Acetyl Sulfisoxazole

Dosage Form	Strength	Route
Tablet	Available in one strength only	Oral
Syrup	Available in one strength only	Oral
Pediatric suspension	Available in one strength only	Oral

When Prescribed: Gantrisin is prescribed for the same reasons as Gantanol. Gantrisin and Gantanol are closely related sulfonamide drugs which kill bacteria. Gantrisin is faster acting but does not reach as high an effective dose. Whether Gantrisin or Gantanol is prescribed depends on the exact nature of the infection.

Precautions and Warnings: See Gantanol.

Side Effects and Adverse Reactions: See Gantanol.

GARAMYCIN CREAM (Schering Corporation)

Generic Name: Gentamicin sulfate

Dosage Form	Strength	Route
Cream	0.1%	Topical (apply directly to affected area)
Ointment	0.1%	Topical

When Prescribed: Garamycin is prescribed for a wide variety of bacterial skin infections. Whether the cream or ointment is prescribed depends on the nature of the infection.

Precautions and Warnings: Garamycin is not effective against fungal infections. Occasionally fungal infections can occur in the same area being treated with Garamycin.

Side Effects and Adverse Reactions: Irritation of skin, itching.

GYNE-LOTRIMIN (Schering Corporation)

Generic Name: Clotrimazole

Dosage Form	Strength	Route
Cream	1%	Intravaginal
Vaginal Tablet	100 mg	Intravaginal

When Prescribed: Gyne-Lotrimin is prescribed for certain infections of the vagina commonly known as yeast infections.

Precautions and Warnings: If relief is not evident in seven to fourteen days, see your physician again.

Side Effects and Adverse Reactions: Vaginal burning, irritation, painful urination.

HALDOL (McNeil Laboratories)

Generic Name: Haloperidol

Dosage Form	Strength	Route
Tablet	0.5 mg	Oral
	1.0 mg	Oral
	2.0 mg	Oral
	5.0 mg	Oral
	10 mg	Oral
Liquid	Available in one strength only	Oral

When Prescribed: Haldol is prescribed for the management of certain emotional disorders. It is often prescribed for extremely hyperactive children.

Precautions and Warnings: If drowsiness occurs you should not drive or operate dangerous machinery. This drug should not be taken with alcohol. Nursing mothers should not use this drug.

Side Effects and Adverse Reactions: Tremors, stiffness, abnormal jerky movements, involuntary movements of tongue, face, mouth, or jaw, insomnia, restlessness, anxiety, mood alterations, agitation, drowsiness, lethargy, headache, confusion, loss of balance, seizures, hallucinations, rapid heart beat, yellowing of the skin, rash, loss of hair, increased sensitivity to sunlight, changes in sex drive, menstrual disorders, breast enlargement, impotence, loss of appetite, constipation, diarrhea, excessive salivation, nausea, vomiting, indigestion, dry mouth, blurred vision, urinary difficulties, breathing difficulties.

HYCOMINE® SYRUP (Endo Laboratories)

Generic Name: Hydrocodone bitartrate, phenylpropanolamine hydrochloride

Dosage Form	Strength	Route
Liquid	Available in one strength only	Oral

When Prescribed: Hycomine is prescribed to control cough and provide relief of congestion in the upper respiratory tract due to the common cold and other ailments.

Precautions and Warnings: Hycomine contains a narcotic which may be habit forming. Patients should not drive or operate machinery while taking this medication.

Side Effects and Adverse Reactions: Drowsiness, heart flutters, dizziness, nervousness, gastrointestinal upset.

HYDERGINE® (Sandoz Pharmaceuticals)

Generic Name: Dihydroergocornine mesylate, dihydroergocristine mesylate, dihydroergokryptine mesylate

Dosage Form	Strength	Route
Tablet	0.5 mg 1.0 mg	sublingual (dissolve under tongue)
Tablet	0.5 mg 1.0 mg	Oral Oral

When Prescribed: Hydergine is prescribed for elderly patients to help reduce some of the symptoms that can accompany old age such as depression, confusion, unsociability, dizziness; and is used to treat migraine headaches.

Precautions and Warnings: Hydergine should be taken under close supervision of your physician.

Side Effects and Adverse Reactions: Irritation under tongue, transient nausea, stomach upset.

HYDROCHLOROTHIAZIDE The generic name for a drug produced by numerous companies in various forms and strengths. Also marketed as:
ORETIC®, Abbott;
ESIDREX®, Ciba;
HYDRODIORIL®, Merck Sharp and Dohme;
THIURETIC®, Parke, Davis & Co.

Generic Name: Hydrochlorothiazide

Dosage Form	Strength	Route
Tablet	25 mg	Oral
	50 mg	Oral
	100 mg	Oral

When Prescribed: Hydrochlorothiazide is prescribed for treatment of high blood pressure or for treatment of water accumulation due to congestive heart failure, cirrhosis of the liver, kidney disease, or other conditions in which water retention is a problem. Hydrochlorothiazide helps the kidneys to pass water and salt.

Precautions and Warnings: This is a potent drug. Frequent check-ups by your physician are required during hydrochlorothiazide therapy. This drug should not be taken by nursing mothers.

Side Effects and Adverse Reactions: Dryness of mouth, thirst, weakness, lethargy, drowsiness, restlessness, muscle pains or cramps, muscular fatigue, urinary disturbances, rapid heart beat, loss of appetite, stomach irritation, nausea, vomiting, stomach cramps, diarrhea, constipation, dizziness, loss of balance, numbness or tingling of skin, headache, yellow appearance of objects, rash, hives, itching.

HYDRODIURIL® (Merck Sharp and Dohme)

Generic Name: Hydrochlorothiazide

Dosage Form	Strength	Route
Tablet	25 mg	Oral
	50 mg*	Oral
	100 mg	Oral

When Prescribed: Hydrodiuril helps the body to pass excess water and salt. It is often prescribed in cases of heart disease, liver problems, kidney disease. Hydrodiuril is also prescribed for high blood pressure.

Precautions and Warnings: Mothers should not nurse while taking this drug.

Side Effects and Adverse Reactions: Loss of appetite, stomach irritation, nausea, vomiting, cramps, diarrhea, constipation, dizziness, loss of balance, numbness, pain or tingling in hands, headache, yellow appearance of objects, faintness, rash, hives, fevers, respiratory distress, sensitivity to sunlight, muscle spasms, weakness, restlessness, transient blurred vision.

HYDROPRES® (Merck Sharp and Dohme)

Generic Name: Hydrochlorothiazide, reserpine

Dosage Form	Strength	Route
Tablet	25 mg	Oral
	50 mg*	Oral

When Prescribed: Hydropres is a combination of two drugs prescribed for the control of high blood pressure. Hydropres is usually not prescribed initially after a diagnosis of high blood pressure, but only after your physician has determined that the fixed combination of drugs in Hydropres is the proper dosage for you.

Precautions and Warnings: Hydropres therapy requires close supervision by your physician. If Hydropres is prescribed for nursing mothers they should discontinue nursing.

Side Effects and Adverse Reactions: Loss of appetite, stomach irritation, nausea, vomiting, cramping, diarrhea, constipation, dizziness, numbness or tingling skin, headache, blurred vision, yellowing of skin, rash, muscle spasm, weakness, restlessness, nightmares, nasal congestion, dryness of mouth, depression, decreased sex drive, rash, hives, heart flutters, sedation, fainting, nervousness, anxiety, increased salivation.

HYGROTON® (USV Laboratories Inc.)

Generic Name: Chlorthalidone

Dosage Form	Strength	Route
Tablet	25 mg	Oral
	50 mg	Oral
	100 mg*	Oral

When Prescribed: Hygroton helps the body pass excess water and salt and is prescribed for use in management of high blood pressure. It may also be prescribed, along with other drugs, for heart disease, liver problems, kidney disorders and during pregnancy.

Precautions and Warnings: Mothers should not nurse while taking this drug.

Side Effects and Adverse Reactions: Dryness of mouth, thirst, weakness, lethargy, drowsiness, restlessness, muscle pains or cramps, muscle fatigue, low blood pressure, frequent urination, rapid heartbeat, nausea, vomiting, loss of appetite, diarrhea, constipation, yellowing of skin or eyes, gastrointestinal distress, dizziness, numbness, headache, yellow appearance of objects, anemia, rash, hives, increased sensitivity to sunlight, fever, respiratory distress, blurred vision, upset stomach, intestinal cramps, impotence.

ILOSONE® (Dista Products Division of Eli Lilly and Company)

Generic Name: Erythromycin estolate

Dosage Form	Strength	Route
Liquid	125 mg/5 ml	Oral
	250 mg/5 ml	Oral
Capsule	125 mg	Oral
(Pulvules®)	250 mg*	Oral
Tablet	250 mg	Oral
	500 mg	Oral
Tablets	125 mg	Oral
(chewable)	250 mg	Oral
Drops	100 .mg/1 ml	Oral

When Prescribed: Ilosone is prescribed for a wide variety of infections. It is often prescribed for infections where penicillin would normally be the drug of choice but the patient has a sensitivity to penicillin.

Precautions and Warnings: Ilosone is an antibiotic which can cause an allergic reaction in susceptible individuals. Serious liver complications have been reported with Ilosone use. This may be accompanied by a general poor feeling, nausea, vomiting, fever or abdominal distress. Patients experiencing any of these symptoms should contact a physician immediately.

Side Effects and Adverse Reactions: The most frequent side effects of erythromycin preparations are gastrointestinal, such as abdominal cramping, discomfort, nausea, vomiting and diarrhea. Other reactions include super-infection by nonsusceptible organisms, hives, rash, fainting, fever, jaundice.

INDERAL® (Ayerst Laboratories)

Generic Name: Propranolol hydrochloride

Dosage Form	Strength	Route
Tablet	10 mg*	Oral
	20 mg	Oral
	40 mg	Oral
	80 mg	Oral

When Prescribed: Inderal is a potent drug which is prescribed for various, often serious, heart conditions such as angina pectoris. It is intended to help the heart beat at a normal rhythm. It is also used to control symptoms of certain tumors of the nervous system, for high blood pressure, and for migraine headache.

Precautions and Warnings: Patients using this drug should be closely monitored, and should not abruptly discontinue the drug after long-term use. If any of the side effects listed below appear, your physician should be contacted immediately.

Side Effects and Adverse Reactions: Slow heartbeat, heart failure, low blood pressure, numbness or tingling of the hands, light-headedness, insomnia, lassitude, weakness, fatigue, mental depression, visual disturbances, hallucinations, disorientation, memory loss, changes in emotions, nausea, vomiting, heartburn, cramps, diarrhea, constipation, rash, fever, sore throat, respiratory distress, anemia, loss of hair.

INDOCIN® (Merck Sharp and Dohme)

Generic Name: Indomethacin, MSD

Dosage Form	Strength	Route
Capsule	25 mg*	Oral
	50 mg	Oral

When Prescribed: Indocin is a potent drug prescribed for relief of pain and swelling in various forms of arthritis where less potent drugs are not effective.

Precautions and Warnings: Indocin is not a simple pain reliever. It should be taken only under close supervision of your physician. Indocin is usually not prescribed for children under 14, pregnant women or nursing mothers. In patients who chronically use Indocin periodic eye examinations should be made. Elderly patients are more susceptible to the adverse side reactions. Patients should not drive or operate machinery while taking Indocin. Should be taken with food, immediately after meals or with antacid to minimize gastric upset.

Side Effects and Adverse Reactions: Ulcers, occasional stomach bleeding, abdominal pain, nausea, vomiting, lack of appetite, heartburn, dizziness, headache, diarrhea, blurred vision, yellowing of skin or eyes, anemia, rash, hives, itching, respiratory distress, ringing in the ears, deafness, depression, confusion, convulsions, pain in extremities, drowsiness, lightheadedness, indigestion, constipation, bloating, flatulence, rectal bleeding, rectal pain, sleepiness, anxiety, muscle weakness, involuntary muscle movements, insomnia, confusion, fainting, heart flutters, swelling, weight gain, vaginal bleeding.

IONAMIN® (Pennwalt Pharmaceutical Division)

Generic Name: Phentermine resin

Dosage Form	Strength	Route
Capsule	15 mg	Oral
	30 mg*	Oral

When Prescribed: Ionamin is a nervous system stimulant prescribed for weight reduction in individuals who cannot lose sufficient weight alone. Ionamin is usually prescribed for a short time (a few weeks) during which diet is also controlled.

Precautions and Warnings: Ionamin may have dangerous interactions with other prescription drugs. Ionamin therapy is not a substitute for diet. Prolonged use of this drug can result in dependency and withdrawal symptoms. The safe use of Ionamin during pregnancy has not been established. This drug is not recommended for use in children under 12 years of age. Ionamin may impair your ability to drive or operate dangerous machinery.

Side Effects and Adverse Reactions: Irregular heart beat, excessive stimulation, restlessness, dizziness, insomnia, euphoria, uneasiness, shaking, headache, dryness of mouth, unpleasant taste, diarrhea, constipation, rash, impotence, change in sex drive.

ISOPTO® CARPINE (Alcon)

Generic Name: Pilocarpine HCl

Dosage Form	Strength	Route
Liquid	.25 % .5 % 1 % 1.5 % 2.0 % 3.0 % 4.0 % 5 % 6 % 8 %	intraocular (eye drop)

When Prescribed: Isopto carpine is prescribed for patients with glaucoma (elevated fluid pressure in eye). It lowers pressure by helping the fluid pass from the eye. It may also be prescribed for other eye disorders.

Precautions and Warnings: To prevent contamination of solution, do not touch eyelids or surrounding area with dropper tip.

Side Effects and Adverse Reactions: Pain in eyes, change in focus, poor vision under conditions of poor illumination.

ISORDIL® (Ives Laboratories)

Generic Name: Isosorbide dinitrate

Dosage Form	Strength	Route
Sublingual tablet	2.5 mg	Dissolve under tongue
	5 mg	Dissolve under tongue
Chewable tablet	10 mg	Oral
Titradose (scored tablet)	5 mg	Oral
	10 mg	Oral
	20 mg	Oral
	30 mg	Oral
Sustained-action tablet	40 mg	Oral
Sustained-action capsule	40 mg	Oral

When Prescribed: Isordil is prescribed for the treatment of pain of coronary artery disease (angina pectoris).

Precautions and Warnings: Patients can develop a tolerance to this drug, which means that more of the drug is necessary to accomplish pain relief. The use of alcohol with this drug may cause adverse reactions.

Side Effects and Adverse Reactions: Flushing, severe persistent headache, dizziness, weakness, nausea, vomiting, restlessness, paleness, perspiration, collapse, rash, skin eruptions.

ISUPREL® MISTOMETER®

(Breon Laboratories Inc.)

Generic Name: Isoproterenol hydrochloride

Dosage Form	Strength	Route
Mist	Available in one strength only	Oral inhalation

When Prescribed: The Isuprel Mistometer is a self-contained unit containing a drug that expands airways in the lungs. It is used for treatment of asthma, emphysema or bronchitis.

Precautions and Warnings: A single dose of mist is usually sufficient for controlling isolated attacks of asthma. Any patient who requires more than three aerosol treatments in a 24-hour period should be under the close supervision of his physician. The mist contains alcohol. This drug may lose its effectiveness if overused.

Side Effects and Adverse Reactions: Throat irritation, rapid, irregular heartbeat, nervousness, nausea, vomiting, headache, flushing of the skin, tremor, dizziness, weakness, sweating, heart pain.

KEFLEX® (Eli Lilly and Company)

Generic Name: Cephalexin monohydrate

Dosage Form	Strength	Route
Capsule	250 mg*	Oral
(Pulvules®)	500 mg	Oral
Liquid	125 mg/5 ml	Oral
	250 mg/5 cc	Oral

When Prescribed: Keflex is an antibiotic prescribed for a variety of infections including those of the respiratory tract, the ear, bone, the skin, and the urogenital tract (including infection of the prostate).

Precautions and Warnings: Allergic reactions to Keflex can occur. People who are allergic to penicillin are often allergic to Keflex. Consult your physician if any side effect or adverse reaction occurs. Safety of Keflex during pregnancy has not been established.

Side Effects and Adverse Reactions: Diarrhea, nausea, vomiting, indigestion, abdominal pain, rash, hives, swelling, itching and infection of the urogenital region, dizziness, fatigue, headache, super-infection by nonsusceptible organisms.

KENALOG® (E. R. Squibb and Sons)

Generic Name: Triamcinolone acetonide

Dosage Form	Strength	Route
Cream	0.025%	Each form
	0.1 %*	is applied
	0.5 %	topically
Lotion	0.025%	to affected
	0.1 %	area
Ointment	0.025%	
	0.1 %	
	0.5 %	
Spray	Available in one strength only	

When Prescribed: Kenalog is a potent drug which is prescribed for topical use for relief of pain, itching, swelling and inflammation caused by various conditions such as allergic reactions.

Precautions and Warnings: Should be kept out of eyes. Kenalog should not be used extensively over large areas of the body or for extended periods of time by pregnant women.

Side Effects and Adverse Reactions: Burning, itching, irritation, dryness, hair follicle infection, excessive hair growth, acnelike eruptions, loss of skin color, dead skin, infection, loss of skin.

K-LYTE/CL (Mead Johnson Pharmaceutical)

Generic Name: Potassium chloride

Dosage Form	Strength	Route
Tablet	Available in one strength only	Oral
Powder	Available in one strength only	Oral

When Prescribed: K-Lyte/Cl is prescribed to replace potassium, an essential salt, in patients who are deficient in potassium. Potassium deficiency can result from the use of drugs that control blood pressure and for other reasons, among which is prolonged diarrhea resulting from a variety of disorders.

Precautions and Warnings: The tablet or the powder must be dissolved completely in the recommended amount of water. K-Lyte/Cl should be taken with meals and sipped slowly over a five to ten minute period.

Side Effects and Adverse Reactions: Nausea, vomiting, diarrhea, abdominal discomfort.

KWELL (Reed and Carnrick)

Generic Name: Gamma benzene hexachloride

Dosage Form	Strength	Route
Cream	Available in one strength only	is applied directly to affected area
Shampoo	Available in one strength only	Topical, each form
Lotion	Available in one strength only	

When Prescribed: Kwell is a drug which kills parasites that live on humans. It is used for the treatment of scabies, a parasitic infection characterized by intense itching especially at night, as well as lice which live in hair on the head and in the pubic region.

Precautions and Warnings: Prolonged or repeated applications should be avoided. Avoid contact with eyes.

Side Effects and Adverse Reactions: Irritation, rash.

LANOXIN® (Burroughs Wellcome)

Generic Name: Digoxin

Dosage Form	Strength	Route
Tablet	0.125 mg	Oral
	0.25 mg*	Oral
	0.5 mg	Oral
Liquid	0.05 mg/cc	Oral

When Prescribed: Lanoxin is a drug which increases the strength of the contractions of the heart. It is prescribed for patients with various forms of heart disease. It may also be used to control an irregular heart beat.

Precautions and Warnings: Lanoxin is a potent drug which can cause serious side effects, particularly if taken in excess. Lanoxin should be taken only under the close supervision of a physician to whom any side effects or adverse reactions should be reported.

Side Effects and Adverse Reactions: Loss of appetite, excessive salivation, nausea, vomiting, diarrhea, lethargy, drowsiness, confusion, visual disturbances, irregular heart beat, blurred vision, changes in color perceptions, headache, weakness.

LAROTID® (Roche Laboratories)

Generic Name: Amoxicillin

Dosage Form	Strength	Route
Capsules	250 mg	Oral
Liquid	125 mg/5 ml	Oral
	250 mg/5 ml	Oral
Pediatric drops	50 mg/1 ml	Oral

When Prescribed: Larotid is a semi-synthetic antibiotic, an analog of ampicillin which is a type of penicillin. Larotid is effective in a wide variety of infections.

Precautions and Warnings: Larotid should not be taken by people who are allergic to penicillin. The use of any penicillin should be discontinued and your physician notified if any of the side effects or reactions listed below appear.

Side Effects and Adverse Reactions: Nausea, vomiting, diarrhea, chest or stomach pains, hypersensitivity reactions such as skin rash, hives, chills, fever, swelling, pain in joints, fainting, super-infection by nonsusceptible organisms, anemia, bruising, darkening of urine.

LASIX® (Hoechst-Roussel Pharmaceuticals Inc.)

Generic Name: Furosemide

Dosage Form	Strength	Route
Tablet	20 mg	Oral
	40 mg*	Oral
Liquid	10 mg/ml	Oral

When Prescribed: Lasix is a potent drug which helps the body to pass excess water and salt, causing a prompt and copious flow of urine. It is used in treatment of heart disease, liver problems, kidney disease and high blood pressure. It is used where weaker agents are deemed not as effective.

Precautions and Warnings: Lasix is not recommended for pregnant women nor for children. Lasix should be taken only under the close supervision of your physician.

Side Effects and Adverse Reactions: Abdominal pain or distension, nausea, vomiting, weakness, fatigue, dizziness, lethargy, leg cramps, loss of appetite, mental confusion, hives, itching, skin reactions, numbness, tingling of skin, blurring of vision, diarrhea, anemia, ringing in the ears, deafness, sweet taste, oral or gastric burning, swelling, headache, yellowing of skin or eyes, blood clots, thirst, increased perspiration, urinary frequency.

LIBRAX® (Roche Products, Inc.)

Generic Name: Chlordiazepoxide hydrochloride, clidinium bromide

Dosage Form	Strength	Route
Capsule	Available in one strength only	Oral

When Prescribed: Librax is prescribed for the relief of symptoms of an overactive gastrointestinal tract and the anxiety and tension that often accompany such disorders. It is often used, along with other drugs, in the management of ulcers.

Precautions and Warnings: Librax should not be taken with alcohol, sedatives, sleeping pills or tranquilizers. Patients using this drug should not drive or operate dangerous machinery. A physical and/or psychological dependence can occur with overuse. The use of this drug during pregnancy should almost always be avoided.

Side Effects and Adverse Reactions: Drowsiness, loss of balance, confusion, fainting, skin eruptions, swelling, menstrual irregularities, nausea, constipation, changes in sex drive, anemia, dryness of mouth, blurring of vision, difficulty in urination.

LIBRIUM® (Roche Products, Inc.)

Generic Name: Chlordiazepoxide hydrochloride

Dosage Form	Strength	Route
Capsule	5 mg	Oral
	10 mg*	Oral
	25 mg	Oral
Libritab® Tablet	5 mg	Oral
	10 mg	Oral
	25 mg	Oral

When Prescribed: Librium is prescribed for a variety of emotional disorders including anxiety, tension and withdrawal symptoms of acute alcoholism. It is also prescribed to relieve the apprehension and anxiety associated with diseases.

Precautions and Warnings: Should not be combined with alcohol, sedatives, tranquilizers or sleeping pills. Persons using this drug should not drive or operate machinery. Physical and/or psychological dependence can occur with overuse. The use of Librium in pregnant women should almost always be avoided.

Side Effects and Adverse Reactions: Drowsiness, loss of balance, confusion, fainting, skin disorders, swelling, menstrual irregularities, nausea, constipation, altered sex drive, fainting, personality changes.

LIDEX® (Syntex Laboratories Inc.)

Generic Name: Fluocinonide

Dosage Form	Strength	Route
Cream	0.05%	Topical (apply directly to affected area)
Ointment	0.05%	Topical (apply directly to affected area)

When Prescribed: Lidex is prescribed for the relief of inflammation, swelling, and itching resulting from various skin disorders.

Precautions and Warnings: Lidex is not for use in the eye. This preparation should not be used extensively by pregnant patients, in large amounts or for prolonged periods of time.

Side Effects and Adverse Reactions: Burning sensation, itching, dryness, infection of skin or hair follicles, skin eruptions, loss of pigment, skin damage.

LOMOTIL® (Searle and Company)

Generic Name: Diphenoxylate hydrochloride, atropine sulfate

Dosage Form	Strength	Route
Tablet	Available in one strength only	Oral
Liquid	Available in one strength only	Oral

When Prescribed: Lomotil is prescribed for the control of diarrhea. It acts by reducing intestinal movements.

Precautions and Warnings: Lomotil is not recommended for pregnant women, nursing mothers or children under the age of 2. Patients using Lomotil should not use alcohol, tranquilizers, sleeping pills or sedatives. This drug can be habit forming if overused.

Side Effects and Adverse Reactions: Dryness of mouth, dryness of skin, inability to urinate, flushing of skin, rash, abdominal discomfort, swelling of the gums, blurred vision, respiratory depression, numbness of the extremities, nausea, sedation, vomiting, headache, dizziness, drowsiness, restlessness, hives, depression, coma, lethargy, loss of appetite, euphoria, itching.

LO/OVRAL® (Wyeth Laboratories)

Generic Name: Norgestrel, ethinyl estradiol

Dosage Form	Strength	Route
Tablet	Available in one strength only	Oral

When Prescribed: Lo/Ovral is an oral contraceptive which contains the same combination of estrogen and progesterone as Ovral and other birth control pills but at a reduced dosage.

Precautions and Warnings: Oral contraceptives are powerful and effective drugs which can have serious side effects including blood clots, strokes, heart attacks, liver tumors, gall bladder disease, and high blood pressure. Safe use of this drug requires a discussion with your physician. A booklet has been prepared to provide you with additional information. Ask your doctor for this booklet. If any of the symptoms listed below are noticed, or anything unusual occurs, consult your physician immediately. Cigarette smoking greatly increases the risk of cardiovascular side effects. Women who use this drug should not smoke.

Side Effects and Adverse Reactions: Nausea, vomiting, abdominal cramps, bloating, bleeding or spotting at times other than during menstruation, change in menstrual flow, pain associated with menstruation, absence of menstruation, temporary infertility after discontinuing treatment, swelling, abnormal darkening of the skin, breast changes, including tenderness, enlargement, and secretion, increase or decrease in body weight, change in vaginal secretions, reduction in amount

LOPRESSOR (Geigy Pharmaceuticals)

Generic Name: Metoprolol tartrate

Dosage Form	Strength	Route
Tablets	50 mg	Oral
	100 mg	Oral

When Prescribed: Lopressor is prescribed to control high blood pressure. It acts directly on the heart to reduce heart rate and blood pressure. It may be prescribed in combination with other drugs for the reduction of blood pressure.

Precautions and Warnings: This drug should not be taken by nursing mothers.

Side Effects and Adverse Reactions: Tiredness, dizziness, depression, headache, nightmares, insomnia, shortness of breath, slow heartbeat, cold extremities, heart flutters, diarrhea, wheezing, nausea, gastric pain, constipation, gas, heartburn, itching, rash, loss of hair, visual disturbances, sore throat, hallucinations, bruising.

Lo/Ovral (Continued)

of breast milk if taken after childbirth, yellowing of skin or eyes, headaches, rash, depression, vaginal infections, cramps, difficulty with contact lenses, visual difficulties, uncontrollable body movements, change in sex drive, change in appetite, nervousness, dizziness, increase of facial hair, loss of scalp hair, itching, skin eruptions.

74

LOTRIMIN (Schering Corporation)

Generic Name: Clotrimazole

Dosage Form	Strength	Route
Cream	1%	Topical (apply directly to the affected area)
Solution	1%	Topical (apply directly to the affected area)

When Prescribed: Lotrimin is an antifungal agent prescribed to treat skin infections caused by various fungal agents.

Precautions and Warnings: This preparation is not intended for use in the eye.

Side Effects and Adverse Reactions: Reddening of the skin, stinging, blistering, peeling, swelling, itching, rash, irritation.

MACRODANTIN® (Norwich-Eaton Pharmaceuticals)

Generic Name: Nitrofurantoin macrocrystals

Dosage Form	Strength	Route
Capsule	25 mg	Oral
	50 mg*	Oral
	100 mg	Oral

When Prescribed: Macrodantin is an antibacterial agent for specific urinary tract infections of the kidney and bladder.

Precautions and Warnings: Macrodantin usually is not prescribed for pregnant women at term or for lactating mothers.

Side Effects and Adverse Reactions: Loss of appetite, nausea, vomiting, diarrhea, cutaneous eruptions, rash, itching, swelling, anemia, chills, fever, yellowing of the skin or eyes, fainting, chest congestion, headache, dizziness, abnormal eye movements, loss of balance, drowsiness, depression, muscle aches, loss of hair, super-infection by nonsusceptible organisms.

MANDELAMINE® (Parke-Davis)

Generic Name: Methenamine mandelate

Dosage Form	Strength	Route
Tablet	250 mg	Oral
	500 mg	Oral
	1000 mg	Oral
Liquid	250 mg/5 ml	Oral
	500 mg/5 ml	Oral

When Prescribed: Mandelamine is prescribed for the management of recurring urinary tract infections. It kills bacteria in the urine.

Precautions and Warnings: Mandelamine is a relatively safe drug that can be used for long-term therapy. However, if overused, painful or difficult urination may result. Your physician may ask you to modify your diet while taking this drug.

Side Effects and Adverse Reactions: Gastrointestinal disturbances, skin rash, difficult or painful urination, superinfection by nonsusceptible organisms.

MARAX® (Roerig)

Generic Name: Ephedrine sulfate, theophylline, hydroxyzine HCl, (alcohol in syrup only)

Dosage Form	Strength	Route
Tablet	Available in one strength only	Oral
Syrup	Available in one strength only	Oral

When Prescribed: Marax is a combination of drugs designed to provide relief of symptoms from bronchial asthma and other bronchial disorders.

Precautions and Warnings: Marax is not recommended for use during early pregnancy. If drowsiness occurs you should not drive or operate dangerous machinery. The possibility of side effects is less if Marax is taken after meals.

Side Effects and Adverse Reactions: Excitation, shaking, insomnia, nervousness, heart flutter, chest pains, dizziness, dryness of nose and throat, headache, sweating, warmth, difficulty in urinating, stomach pains, heartburn, nausea, vomiting, frequent urination, drowsiness.

MEDROL® (The Upjohn Company)

Generic Name: Methylprednisolone

Dosage Form	Strength	Route
Tablet	2 mg	Oral
	4 mg	Oral
	8 mg	Oral
	16 mg	Oral
	24 mg	Oral
	32 mg	Oral
Dosepak™	4 mg*	Oral

When Prescribed: Medrol is the manmade equivalent of a substance produced naturally in the body by the adrenal glands. The main action of Medrol is to reduce inflammation and swelling. Medrol is prescribed for a variety of reasons including glandular disorders, rheumatic and arthritic disorders, diseases of connective tissues, skin diseases, allergies, eye disorders, respiratory diseases, blood disorders, swelling, meningitis, tuberculosis, gastrointestinal diseases, swelling from dental work.

Precautions and Warnings: Mothers taking Medrol should not nurse. Patients on Medrol therapy should not receive smallpox or other vaccinations. Prolonged use of Medrol may cause psychological and/or physical dependence and subsequent withdrawal symptoms.

Side Effects and Adverse Reactions: Fluid retention, swelling, muscle weakness, ulcer, stomach irritation, slow wound healing, increased sweating, allergic skin reactions, convulsions, dizziness, headache, menstrual irregularities, suppression of growth in children, bulging of the eyes.

MELLARIL® (Sandoz Pharmaceuticals)

Generic Name: Thioridazine hydrochloride

Dosage Form	Strength	Route
Tablet	10 mg	Oral
	15 mg	Oral
	25 mg*	Oral
	50 mg	Oral
	100 mg	Oral
	150 mg	Oral
	200 mg	Oral
Liquid	30 mg/ml	Oral
	100 mg/ml	Oral

When Prescribed: Mellaril is prescribed for management of certain emotional disorders which are characterized by abnormal agitation, aggressiveness or excitement. It is often prescribed for overaggressive children. It can also be prescribed for use in alcohol withdrawal, severe pain and senility.

Precautions and Warnings: This drug may impair mental and/or physical abilities required for performance of hazardous tasks such as operating machinery or driving motor vehicles. Mellaril should not be taken with alcohol, tranquilizers, sleeping pills or sedatives.

Side Effects and Adverse Reactions: Drowsiness, uncoordinated movements, tremors, confusion, hyperactivity, lethargy, psychotic reactions, rest-

(Continued on page 78)

Mellaril (Continued)

lessness, headache, dryness of mouth, blurred vision, constipation, nausea, vomiting, diarrhea, nasal stuffiness, paleness, breast enlargement, lack of menstruation, inhibition of ejaculation, false positive pregnancy tests, swelling, skin eruptions, hives, loss of appetite, anemia, fever, yellowing of skin or eyes, heart failure, abnormal movements of the face, tongue or jaws, loss of visual acuity, brownish coloring of vision, impairment of night vision, urinary difficulties.

Meprobamate (Continued)

the heart, increased heart rate, fainting, itching, rash, hives, anemia, swelling, fever, chills, frequent urination, inability to urinate, darkening of urine.

MEPROBAMATE
The generic name for a drug produced by numerous companies in various forms and strengths. Also marketed as:
EQUANIL®, Wyeth;
KESSO–BAMATE®, McKesson;
MEPROSPAN®, Wallace;
MEPROTABS®, Wallace;
MILTOWN®, Wallace;
SK–BAMATE®, Smith Kline and French.

Generic Name: Meprobamate

Dosage Form	Strength	Route
Tablet	200 mg	Oral
	400 mg*	Oral

When Prescribed: Meprobamate is prescribed for the relief of anxiety and tension, often in patients with various disease states which lead to anxiety and tension. It is also used to promote sleep in tense, anxious patients.

Precautions and Warnings: Overuse of this drug can lead to physical and/or psychological dependence. Sudden withdrawal after prolonged and excessive use may cause adverse reactions. Meprobamate may impair the mental or physical abilities required for the performance of potentially hazardous tasks such as driving or operating machinery. Should not be taken with alcohol, tranquilizers, sedatives or sleeping pills. The safe use of this drug in pregnancy has not been established.

Side Effects and Adverse Reactions: Drowsiness, loss of balance, dizziness, slurred speech, headache, weakness, tingling, crawling skin, inability of eyes to adapt to changing light, euphoria, stimulation, excitement, nausea, vomiting, diarrhea, flutters of

78

MINIPRESS (Pfizer Laboratories Division)

Generic Name: Prazosin hydrochloride

Dosage Form	Strength	Route
Capsule	1 mg	Oral
	2 mg	Oral
	5 mg	Oral

When Prescribed: Minipress is prescribed to reduce blood pressure in patients with high blood pressure. It may be prescribed as the sole agent or in combination with other agents for the management of high blood pressure.

Precautions and Warnings: Lowering of blood pressure (the intended effect of the drug) can lead to fainting associated with changes in posture. For example, after getting up from a chair you may experience light-headedness or fainting. This is more likely to occur when Minipress therapy is just starting.

Side Effects and Adverse Reactions: Dizziness, headache, drowsiness, lack of energy, weakness, heart flutters, fainting, nausea, vomiting, diarrhea, constipation, abdominal upset, swelling, breathing difficulties, rapid heartbeat, nervousness, loss of balance, depression, abnormal skin sensation, rash, itching, urinary difficulties, impotence, blurred vision, red eyes, ringing in ears, dry mouth, nasal congestion.

MINOCIN® (Lederle Laboratories)

Generic Name: Minocycline hydrochloride

Dosage Form	Strength	Route
Capsule	50 mg	Oral
	100 mg*	Oral
Syrup	50 mg/5 ml	Oral

When Prescribed: Minocin is a derivative of tetracycline, an effective antibiotic prescribed for many different types of infection. It is often used in place of penicillin in patients who are allergic to penicillin.

Precautions and Warnings: Minocin should not be taken by people overly sensitive to tetracycline. If any of the side effects listed below occur, consult your physician immediately. This drug can interfere with tooth development and therefore is not recommended for pregnant women, infants, or children under the age of 8. Antacids will impair absorption.

Side Effects and Adverse Reactions: Exaggerated sunburn, super-infection by nonsusceptible organisms, loss of appetite, nausea, vomiting, diarrhea, difficulty in swallowing, stomach pains, skin rash, hives, swelling, dizziness, fainting.

MONISTAT® 7 (Ortho Pharmaceuticals)

Generic Name: Miconazole nitrate

Dosage Form	Strength	Route
Cream	Available in one strength only	Intra-vaginal

When Prescribed: Monistat is prescribed for "yeast" (or fungal) infections of the skin and of the mucous membranes of the vagina.

Precautions and Warnings: If irritation or sensitivity occurs discontinue use and consult your physician.

Side Effects and Adverse Reactions: Burning, itching, irritation, pelvic cramps, hives, skin rash, headache.

MOTRIN® (The Upjohn Company)

Generic Name: Ibuprofen

Dosage Form	Strength	Route
Tablet	300 mg	Oral
	400 mg*	Oral
	600 mg	Oral

When Prescribed: Motrin is prescribed to relieve the pain and inflammation of arthritis. Motrin is as effective as aspirin for the long-term management of pain and inflammation but usually is better tolerated in terms of stomach upset and irritation.

Precautions and Warnings: Ingestion of motrin is not recommended during pregnancy, nor for nursing mothers. The use of aspirin with motrin may reduce the effectiveness of the drug.

Adverse Reactions and Side Effects: Nausea, chest pains, heartburn, diarrhea, constipation or gastric pain, abdominal cramps or pain, vomiting, indigestion, constipation, bloating, gas, dizziness, headache, nervousness, rash, ringing in the ears, decreased appetite, depression, insomnia, visual disturbances, nightmares, fever, itching.

MYCOLOG® (E. R. Squibb and Sons)

Generic Name: Nystatin, neomycin sulfate, gramicidin, triamcinolone acetonide

Dosage Form	Strength	Route
Cream and Ointment	Available in one strength only	Applied directly to problem area

When Prescribed: Mycolog is a topical cream that provides rapid, complete, often prolonged control of symptoms of inflammation of the skin, infections of the skin and itching of the skin. Mycolog is a combination of an antifungal agent, antibacterial agents, and a corticosteroid.

Precautions and Warnings: <u>Mycolog should not be used extensively or for prolonged periods in pregnant patients.</u> This preparation is not intended for use in the eyes.

Side Effects and Adverse Reactions: Burning, itching, irritation, dryness, hair follicle infections, excessive hair growth, skin eruptions, loss of pigmentation, peeling or flaking skin, superinfection by nonsusceptible organisms.

MYCOSTATIN® (E. R. Squibb and Sons)

Generic Name: Nystatin

Dosage Form	Strength	Route
Vaginal tablet	Each form is available in one strength only	Intravaginal
Cream		Topical
Ointment		Topical
Tablet		Oral
Liquid		Oral

When Prescribed: Mycostatin is prescribed for the control of fungus (yeast) infections.

Precautions and Warnings: Mycostatin should not be used by patients with a sensitivity to the drug.

Side Effects and Adverse Reactions: Large doses of the oral forms of Mycostatin may produce diarrhea, gastrointestinal distress, nausea, vomiting.

MYSTECLIN F® (E. R. Squibb and Sons)

Generic Name: Tetracycline, amphotericin B, potassium metaphosphate

Dosage Form	Strength	Route
Capsule	Available in one strength only	Oral
Liquid	Available in one strength only	Oral

When Prescribed: Mysteclin F is prescribed for various types of infection including those of the respiratory, gastrointestinal and urogenital systems. It can be used for the treatment of serious acne problems. Amphotericin is present for the prevention of secondary infections that may arise in patients on antibiotic therapy.

Precautions and Warnings: Mysteclin contains tetracycline, which may produce allergic reactions in susceptible individuals. Not recommended for pregnant women, infants or children under the age of 8.

Side Effects and Adverse Reactions: Loss of appetite, heartburn, nausea, vomiting, diarrhea, gastrointestinal problems, itching of rectal area, black hairy tongue, sore throat, difficulty in swallowing, hoarseness, skin rashes, exaggerated sunburn, hives, fever, aching joints, fainting, anemia, superinfection by nonsusceptible organisms.

NALDECON® (Bristol Laboratories)

Generic Name: Phenylpropanolamine hydrochloride, phenylephrine hydrochloride, phenyltoloxamine citrate, chlorpheniramine maleate

Dosage Form	Strength	Route
Table	Available in one strength only	Oral
Liquid	Available in one strength only	Oral
Pediatric drops	Available in one strength only	Oral
Pediatric syrup	Available in one strength only	Oral

When Prescribed: Naldecon is prescribed for the relief of symptoms of colds and other upper respiratory infections, sinus infections, hay fever and allergies.

Precautions and Warnings: This drug may cause drowsiness. Do not drive or operate machinery while taking this drug.

Side Effects and Adverse Reactions: Rash, hives, anemia, drowsiness, lassitude, giddiness, dryness of mouth or nose, painful urination, elevated blood pressure, irregular heart beat, headache, faintness, dizziness, ringing in the ears, loss of appetite, nausea, vomiting, diarrhea, constipation.

NALFON (Dista Products Company)

Generic Name: Fenoprofen calcium

Dosage Form	Strength	Route
Capsule	300 mg	Oral
Tablet	600 mg	Oral

When Prescribed: Nalfon is prescribed for the relief of pain and inflammation from arthritis. It is as effective as aspirin in reducing pain and inflammation but is usually better tolerated in the stomach.

Precautions and Warnings: This drug is not recommended for pregnant women or for nursing mothers. Nalfon should be taken thirty minutes before or two hours after a meal.

Side Effects and Adverse Reactions: Indigestion, constipation, nausea, abdominal pain, loss of appetite, blood in stool, diarrhea, gas, dry mouth, itching, rash, increased sweating, hives, sleepiness, dizziness, tremors, confusion, insomnia, ringing in the ears, blurred vision, decreased ability to hear, heart flutters, rapid heartbeat, headache, nervousness, weakness, breathing difficulties, swelling, fatigue, mood depression, urinary difficulties.

NAPROSYN (Syntex Puerto Rico, Inc.)

Generic Name: Naproxen

Dosage Form	Strength	Route
Tablet	250 mg	Oral

When Prescribed: Naprosyn is prescribed for the relief of pain and inflammation from arthritis. It is as effective as aspirin in reducing pain and inflammation but is usually better tolerated in the stomach.

Precautions and Warnings: This drug is not recommended for pregnant women or nursing mothers. If drowsiness occurs you should not drive or operate dangerous machinery.

Side Effects and Adverse Reactions: Heartburn, nausea, indigestion, abdominal pain, constipation, upset stomach, diarrhea, vomiting, blood in stools, headache, drowsiness, dizziness, light-headedness, loss of balance, inability to concentrate, depression, itching, skin eruptions, sweating, rash, hives, ringing in the ears, visual disturbances, hearing disturbances, swelling, heart flutters, breathing difficulties, yellowing of the skin.

NEMBUTAL® SODIUM (Abbott Laboratories)

Generic Name: Sodium pentobarbital

Dosage Form	Strength	Route
Capsule	30 mg	Oral
	50 mg	Oral
	100 mg*	Oral

When Prescribed: Nembutal Sodium is used as a sedative or sleeping pill in cases where weaker drugs are not deemed effective. Nembutal Sodium is a powerful central nervous system depressant.

Precautions and Warnings: This drug may impair mental and/or physical abilities required for performance of hazardous tasks such as driving or operating machinery. Nembutal Sodium should not be taken with alcohol, tranquilizers, sleeping pills or sedatives. This drug may be habit forming. The safe use of Nembutal Sodium in pregnancy has not been established.

Side Effects and Adverse Reactions: Respiratory depression, depressed breathing rate, coma, heart failure, skin rash, allergic reactions, drowsiness, lethargy, hangover, nausea, vomiting, excitement.

NEODECADRON® OPHTHALMIC SOLUTION (Merck Sharp and Dohme)

Generic Name: Dexamethasone sodium phosphate, neomycin

Dosage Form	Strength	Route
Liquid	Available in one strength only	Eyedrops

When Prescribed: Neodecadron ophthalmic solution is a potent drug which is prescribed for treatment of inflammation of the eye and surrounding tissue. It is effective in reducing inflammation often associated with infection. This preparation contains a steroid to reduce inflammation and an antibiotic, as well.

Precautions and Warnings: If used for prolonged periods, eye examinations should be performed frequently. This preparation should not be used for prolonged periods by pregnant patients.

Side Effects and Adverse Reactions: Increased eye pressure, nerve damage, visual defects, cataracts, secondary infection, stinging, burning.

NEOSPORIN® OPHTHALMIC SOLUTION (Burroughs Wellcome Company)

Generic Name: Polymyxin B–Neomycin Gramicidin

Dosage Form	Strength	Route
Liquid	Available in one strength only	Eyedrops

When Prescribed: Neosporin is prescribed for the short-term treatment of superficial infections of the eye.

Precautions and Warnings: The solution as contained in the bottle is sterile. Patients should use caution in placing the drops into the eye so as to not contaminate the dropper. This is best done by preventing the tip from touching the eyelid or surrounding areas.

Side Effects and Adverse Reactions: Sensitization of the skin or surface of the eye.

NICOTINIC ACID (The generic name of a drug produced by numerous companies in various forms and strengths. Also marked as: NICOBID®, Armour; SK–NIACIN®, Smith Kline and French; NICO–400®, Marion; NICOTINEX®, Fleming.

Generic Name: Nicotinic acid (also known as niacin)

Dosage Form	Strength	Route
Capsule	125 mg	Oral
	250 mg	Oral
Tablets	500 mg	Oral

When Prescribed: Nicotinic acid (niacin) is a vitamin, necessary for normal body function. In larger doses it can reduce serum lipids (fat and cholesterol in the blood).

Precautions and Warnings: The safety of high doses of nicotinic acid for pregnant or nursing mothers has not been established.

Side Effects and Adverse Reactions: Flushing, feeling of warmth, stomach disturbances, dryness of the skin, itching or tingling of skin, rash, allergies, headaches.

NITRO-BID® (Marion Laboratories, Inc.)

Generic Name: Nitroglycerin

Dosage Form	Strength	Route
Capsule	2.5 mg	Oral
(plateau	6.5 mg	Oral
capsule®)	9.0 mg	Oral
prolonged action		

When Prescribed: Nitro-Bid is prescribed for the relief of angina pectoris (chest pain) which often accompanies heart conditions such as coronary artery disease. It acts by increasing the blood flow to the heart muscle.

Precautions and Warnings: While some nitroglycerin preparations are meant to be dissolved under the tongue, Nitro-bid capsules should be swallowed. Nitro-bid is not intended for immediate relief of angina attacks but meant to produce relief for 8 to 12 hours.

Side Effects and Adverse Reactions: Severe and persistent headaches, cutaneous flushing, dizziness, weakness, nausea, vomiting, rash. Adverse reactions are made worse if alcohol is consumed.

NITROGLYCERIN: The generic name for a drug produced by numerous companies in various forms and strengths. Also marked as:
NITROBID®, Marion;
NITROBON®, Forest;
0.4 mg* NITROSPAN®, USV Pharmaceuticals;
NITROL®, Kremers-Urban Co.;
NITROSTAT®, Parke Davis & Co.

See NITRO-BID or NITROSTAT

NITROSTAT (Parke-Davis)

Generic Name: Nitroglycerin

Dosage Form	Strength	Route
Tablet	0.15	Sublingual (dissolve under tongue)
	0.3	Sublingual
	0.4	Sublingual
	0.6	Sublingual

When Prescribed: Nitrostat is prescribed for the relief of attacks of angina pectoris that are often present in various forms of heart disease. This preparation increases the blood flow to the heart muscle.

Precautions and Warnings: Nitrostat should be dissolved under the tongue or between the gum and cheek. Do not swallow the tablet. If blurred vision or dryness of mouth occurs discontinue and consult your physician.

Side Effects and Adverse Reactions: Blurred vision, dryness of mouth, transient headache, loss of balance, weakness, heart flutters, fainting.

NOLUDAR® (Roche Laboratories)

Generic Name: Methyprylon

Dosage Form	Strength	Route
Capsule	300 mg	Oral
Tablet	50 mg	Oral
	200 mg	Oral

When Prescribed: Noludar is prescribed as a sleeping pill for relief of insomnia due to a variety of reasons.

Precautions and Warnings: Patients should not drive or operate machinery after taking this drug. Noludar should not be taken with alcohol, tranquilizers, sedatives or other sleeping pills. Overuse of Noludar can cause physical and/or psychological dependence.

Side Effects and Adverse Reactions: Morning drowsiness, dizziness, diarrhea, heartburn, nausea, vomiting, headache, excitation, skin rash. Abrupt withdrawal of Noludar may cause convulsions.

NORGESIC® (Riker Laboratories, Inc.)

Generic Name: Orphenadrine citrate, aspirin, phenacetin, caffeine

Dosage Form	Strength	Route
Tablet	Available in one strength only	Oral

When Prescribed: Norgesic is prescribed for the relief of mild to moderate pain of muscle or skeletal disorders. It is often prescribed for muscle pulls, cramps, sprains. It may also be prescribed to control pain of arthritis, dental procedures, menstruation or minor surgery.

Precautions and Warnings: Since severe adverse reactions can occur when Norgesic is taken with certain pain relievers such as Darvon, you should only take Norgesic with other medication if your physician directs you to do so. The safe use of Norgesic in pregnant women or children has not been established. This drug may impair your ability to drive or operate machinery.

Side Effects and Adverse Reactions: Rapid heart, irregular heart beat, inability to urinate, dry mouth, blurred vision, dilation of pupils, eye pressure, weakness, nausea, vomiting, headache, dizziness, constipation, drowsiness, rash, hives, excitation, confusion, hallucinations, lightheadedness, fainting.

NORINYL® (Syntex [F.P.] Inc.)

Generic Name: Norethindrone, mestranol

Dosage Form	Strength	Route
Tablet	1/50 21	Oral
	1/50 28	Oral
	1/80 21	Oral
	1/80 28	Oral
	2 mg	

When Prescribed: Norinyl is an oral contraceptive. In the 1/50 and 1/80 forms it is prescribed for birth control only. In the 2 mg form it is prescribed for birth control and menstrual irregularities.

Precautions and Warnings: Oral contraceptives are powerful and effective drugs which can have serious side effects including blood clots, strokes, heart attacks, liver tumors, gall bladder disease, and high blood pressure. Safe use of this drug requires a discussion with your physician. A booklet has been prepared to provide you with additional information. Ask your doctor for this booklet. If any of the symptoms listed below are noticed, or anything unusual occurs, consult your physician immediately. Cigarette smoking increases the risk of cardiovascular side effects. Women who use Norinyl should not smoke.

Side Effects and Adverse Reactions: Nausea, vomiting, abdominal cramps, bloating, bleeding or spotting at times other than during menstruation, change in menstrual flow, pain associated with menstruation, absence of menstruation, temporary infertility after discontinuing treatment, swelling, abnormal darkening of the skin,

Norinyl (Continued)

breast changes, including tenderness, enlargement, and secretion, increase or decrease in body weight, change in vaginal secretions, reduction in amount of breast milk if taken after birth, yellowing of skin or eyes, headaches, rash, depression, vaginal infections, cramps, difficulty with contact lenses, visual difficulties, uncontrollable body movements, change in sex drive, change in appetite, nervousness, dizziness, increase of facial hair, loss of scalp hair, itching, skin eruptions.

Norlestrin (Continued)

ginal secretions, reduction in the amount of breast milk if taken after childbirth, yellowing of skin or eyes, headaches, rash, depression, vaginal infections, cramps, difficulties with contact lenses, visual difficulties, uncontrollable body movements, change in sex drive, change in appetite, nervousness, dizziness, increase in facial hair, loss of scalp hair, itching, skin eruptions.

NORLESTRIN® (Parke Davis Laboratories)

Generic Name: Norethindrone acetate, ethinyl estradiol

Dosage Form	Strength		Route
Tablet	1/50	21	Oral
	2.5/50	21	Oral
	1/50	28	Oral
	1/50	Fe	Oral
	2.5/50	Fe	Oral

When Prescribed: Norlestrin is an oral contraceptive. It is prescribed for birth control in all strengths. The 21 strengths are taken for 3 weeks each cycle. The 28 and Fe strengths are taken every day.

Precautions and Adverse Reactions: Oral contraceptives are powerful and effective drugs which can produce serious side effects including blood clots, strokes, heart attacks, liver tumors, gall bladder disease, and high blood pressure. Safe use of this drug requires a discussion with your physician. If any of the symptoms listed below are noticed or anything unusual occurs, consult your physician immediately. Cigarette smoking increases the risk of cardiovascular side effects. Women who use this drug should not smoke.

Side Effects and Adverse Reactions: Nausea, vomiting, abdominal cramps, bloating, bleeding or spotting at times other than during menstruation, change in menstrual flow, pain associated with menstruation, absence of menstruation, temporary infertility after discontinuing treatment, swelling, abnormal darkening of the skin, breast changes including tenderness, enlargement, and secretion, increase or decrease in body weight, change in va-

NOVAHISTINE® DH (Dow Pharmaceuticals)

Generic Name: codeine phosphate, phenylpropanolamine hydrochloride, chlorpheniramine maleate, alcohol

Dosage Form	Strength	Route
Liquid	Available in one strength only	Oral

When Prescribed: Novahistine DH is prescribed for relief from cough and nasal congestion, due to colds or other respiratory infections. It can also be prescribed for relief of congestion in ears.

Precautions and Warnings: Novahistine may interact with other drugs you are taking. This drug may be habit forming. The codeine in Novahistine may potentiate the effects of alcohol, pain relievers, sleeping pills and sedatives. If drowsiness occurs, do not drive or operate machinery.

Side Effects and Adverse Reactions: Nausea, vomiting, constipation, dizziness, sedation, heart flutters, fear, anxiety, tenseness, restlessness, shaking, weakness, pale skin, difficulty in breathing, urinary problems, insomnia, hallucinations, convulsions, itching.

NOVAHISTINE® EXPECTORANT (Dow Pharmaceuticals)

Generic Name: Codeine phosphate, phenylpropanolamine hydrochloride, glyceryl guaiacolate, alcohol

Dosage Form	Strength	Route
Liquid	Available in one strength only	Oral

When Prescribed: Novahistine Expectorant is prescribed to relieve cough and congestion in bronchial disorders. It may also be prescribed for certain ear disorders. This drug acts by reducing the urge to cough, reducing secretions, and dislodging phlegm.

Precautions and Warnings: Novahistine Expectorant contains codeine which may be habit forming. Novahistine Expectorant may have potentially serious interactions with other drugs you may be taking. If drowsiness occurs do not drive or operate dangerous machinery.

Side Effects and Adverse Reactions: Nausea, vomiting, constipation, dizziness, drowsiness, itching, irregular heart beat, fear, anxiety, tension, restlessness, tremors, weakness, respiratory difficulties, pallor, urinary difficulties, insomnia, hallucinations, convulsions, depression.

OMNIPEN® (Wyeth Laboratories)

Generic Name: Ampicillin

Dosage Form	Strength	Route
Capsule	250 mg*	Oral
	500 mg	Oral
Suspension	125 mg/5 ml	Oral
	250 mg/5 ml	Oral

When Prescribed: Omnipen is a semi-synthetic penicillin that is effective in a wide variety of infections.

Precautions and Warnings: Omnipen should not be taken by people who are allergic to penicillin. The use of any penicillin should be discontinued and your physician notified if any of the side effects listed below appear.

Side Effects and Adverse Reactions: Nausea, vomiting, chest or stomach pains, diarrhea, changes in color/texture of tongue and oral mucous membranes, skin rash, hives, chills, fever, swelling, pain in joints, fainting, super-infection by non-susceptible organisms, anemia, abnormal bruising, indigestion, darkening of urine.

ORINASE® (The Upjohn Company)

Generic Name: Tolbutamide

Dosage Form	Strength	Route
Tablet	Available in one strength only	Oral

When Prescribed: Orinase is prescribed for diabetes (diabetes mellitus) of the stable type without complications. This type is known as mild adult diabetes. Orinase is not effective in juvenile diabetes. Orinase is prescribed only after it has been decided that dietary control alone cannot sufficiently control blood sugar. It sometimes is prescribed to replace insulin or to be taken with insulin. Orinase acts by helping the body to release its own insulin.

Precautions and Warnings: Patients are given Orinase only under very strict supervision of the physician. Frequent checkups are necessary. If at any time you do not feel well while taking this drug you should report to your physician immediately. Not recommended for pregnant women.

Side Effects and Adverse Reactions: Hypoglycemia (low blood sugar) and/or skin sensitivity to sunlight can occur as a result of alcohol ingestion among other factors. Other reactions include nausea, chest pains, heartburn, headache, hives, rash, skin eruptions, yellowing of skin or eyes, anemia.

ORNADE® SPANSULES® (Smith Kline and French Laboratories)

Generic Name: Chlorpheniramine maleate, phenylpropanolamine hydrochloride, isopropamide iodide

Dosage Form	Strength	Route
Capsule (Time Release)	Available in one strength only	Oral

When Prescribed: Ornade is prescribed for the relief of sneezing, running nose, watery eyes and nasal congestion associated with the common cold, sinus infections, hay fever and allergies.

Precautions and Warnings: Ornade is not intended for use in children under 6. Patients should not drive or operate machinery while taking this drug. Ornade should not be taken with alcohol, tranquilizers, sleeping pills or sedatives.

Side Effects and Adverse Reactions: Drowsiness, excessive dryness of nose, throat, or mouth, nervousness, insomnia, nausea, vomiting, heartburn, diarrhea, rash, dizziness, weakness, tightness of chest, pain in chest or abdomen, irregular heart beat, headache, tremors, lack of coordination, painful or difficult urination, anemia, convulsions, changes in blood pressure, loss of appetite, constipation, visual disturbances, acne, swollen glands.

ORTHO-NOVUM® (Ortho Pharmaceuticals)

Generic Name: Norethindrone, mestranol

Dosage Form	Strength	Route
Tablet	1/50 21*	Oral
	1/50 28	Oral
	1/80 21*	Oral
	1/80 28	Oral
	2 mg	Oral
	10 mg	Oral

When Prescribed: Ortho-Novum is an oral contraceptive. In the 1/50 and 1/80 forms it is prescribed for birth control only. In the 2 mg and 10 mg form it is prescribed for birth control and menstrual irregularities.

Precautions and Warnings: Oral contraceptives are powerful and effective drugs which can cause serious side effects including blood clots (which may lead to strokes, heart attacks), liver tumors, gall bladder disease, and high blood pressure. Safe use of this drug requires a discussion with your physician. A booklet has been prepared to provide you with additional information. Ask your doctor for this booklet. If any of the symptoms listed below are noticed or anything unusual occurs, consult your physician immediately. Cigarette smoking increases the risk of cardiovascular side effects. Women taking Ortho-Novum should not smoke.

Side Effects and Adverse Reactions: Nausea, vomiting, abdominal cramps, bloating, bleeding or spotting at times other than during menstruation, change in menstrual flow, pain associated with menstruation, absence of menstruation, temporary infertility

Ortho-Novum (Continued)

after discontinuing treatment, swelling, abnormal darkening of the skin, breast changes, including tenderness, enlargement, and secretion, increase or decrease in body weight, changes in vaginal secretions, reduction in amount of breast milk if taken after childbirth, yellowing of skin or eyes, headaches, rash, depression, vaginal infections, cramps, difficulty with contact lenses, visual difficulties, uncontrollable body movements, change in sex drive, change in appetite, dizziness, increase of facial hair, loss of scalp hair, itching, skin eruptions, changes in personality such as nervousness.

Ovral (Continued)

childbirth, yellowing of skin or eyes, headaches, rash, depression, vaginal infections, cramps, difficulty with contact lenses, visual difficulties, uncontrollable body movements, change in sex drive, change in appetite, nervousness, dizziness, increase of facial hair, loss of scalp hair, itching, skin eruptions.

OVRAL® (Wyeth Laboratories)

Generic Name: Norgestrel, ethinyl estradiol

Dosage Form	Strength	Route
Tablet	Available in one strength only	Oral

When Prescribed: Ovral is an oral contraceptive. Like other contraceptives it is a combination of estrogen and progesterone.

Precautions and Warnings: Oral contraceptives are powerful and effective drugs which can have serious side effects including blood clots, strokes, heart attacks, liver tumors, gall bladder disease, and high blood pressure. Safe use of this drug requires a discussion with your physician. A booklet has been prepared to provide you with additional information. Ask your doctor for this booklet. If any of the symptoms listed below are noticed or anything unusual occurs, consult your physician immediately. Cigarette smoking increases the risk of cardiovascular side effects. Women who take Ovral should not smoke.

Side Effects and Adverse Reactions: Nausea, vomiting, abdominal cramps, bloating, bleeding or spotting at times other than during menstruation, change in menstrual flow, pain associated with menstruation, absence of menstruation, temporary infertility after discontinuing treatment, swelling, abnormal darkening of the skin, breast changes, including tenderness, enlargement, and secretion, increase or decrease in body weight, changes in vaginal secretions, reduction in amount of breast milk if taken after

OVULEN–21® (Searle and Company)

Generic Name: Ethynodiol diacetate, mestranol

Dosage Form	Strength	Route
Tablet	Available in one strength only	Oral

When Prescribed: Ovulen is an oral contraceptive combining estrogen and progesterone.

Precautions and Warnings: An increased risk of blood clots and other serious disorders have been associated with the use of hormonal contraceptives such as Ovulen-21. Oral contraceptives should be taken only under the supervision of a physician. A booklet has been prepared to provide you with additional information; ask your physician for it. If any of the symptoms listed below appear, discuss continued use of the drug with a physician. Smoking increases the risk of cardiovascular side effects. Women who use this drug should not smoke.

Side Effects and Adverse Reactions: Nausea, vomiting, stomach cramps, bleeding or spotting at times other than during "period," changes in amount of menstrual flow, absence of menstruation, swelling, abnormal darkening of skin, changes in breasts including tenderness, enlargement, secretion, an increase or decrease in weight, suppression of lactation when taken immediately after childbirth, migraine, rash, rise in blood pressure, mental depression, changes in sex drive, changes in appetite, headache, nervousness, dizziness, fatigue, backache, increase in facial hair, loss of scalp hair, itching.

PANMYCIN® (The Upjohn Company)

Generic Name: Tetracyline hydrochloride

Dosage Form	Strength	Route
Capsule	250 mg	Oral
Syrup	125 mg/5 ml	Oral
Tablets	250 mg	Oral
	500 mg	Oral
Liquid	100 mg/ml	Oral

When Prescribed: Panmycin is an effective antibiotic prescribed for many different types of infection. It is often used in place of penicillin in patients who are allergic to penicillin.

Precautions and Warnings: Panmycin should not be taken by people overly sensitive to tetracycline. If any of the side effects listed below occur, consult your physician immediately. Not recommended for pregnant women, infants or children under the age of 8.

Side Effects and Adverse Reactions: Exaggerated sunburn, super-infection by nonsusceptible organisms, loss of appetite, nausea, vomiting, diarrhea, inflammation of the tongue, difficulty swallowing, stomach pains, inflammation of the bowel and genital regions, skin rash, hives, swelling, shock.

PAPAVERINE HCL: The generic name for a drug produced by numerous companies in various forms and strengths.
Also marketed as:
CEREBID, Saron;
CERESPAN, USV Pharmaceutical;
COPAVIN, Lilly;
P-200, Boots;
PAVABID, Marion;
PAVAKEY, Key Pharmaceuticals;
PAVATRAN, Mayrand;
THERAPAV, Berlex;
VASOSPAN, Ulmer.

Generic Name: Papaverine HCl

Dosage Form	Strength	Route

Available in various forms and strengths for use orally.

When Prescribed: Papaverine HCl is prescribed to relieve spasm of blood vessels in patients with various cardiovascular disorders. It is also prescribed to relieve spasm in patients with various forms of colic.

Precautions and Warnings: If this drug causes drowsiness you should not drive or operate dangerous machinery.

Side Effects and Adverse Reactions: Constipation, general discomfort, flushing, sweating, increase in depth of respiration, increase in heart rate, drowsiness.

PARAFON FORTE® (McNeil Laboratories Inc.)

Generic Name: Chlorzoxazone, acetaminophen

Dosage Form	Strength	Route
Tablet	Available in one strength only	Oral

When Prescribed: Parafon Forte is prescribed for the relief of pain and stiffness of muscle and bone disorders. It is often prescribed for chronic muscle spasm.

Precautions and Warnings: The safe use of this drug in pregnancy has not been established.

Side Effects and Adverse Reactions: Gastrointestinal disturbances, drowsiness, dizziness, light-headedness, depression, stimulation, rashes, discoloration of urine, skin eruptions, hives.

PAREGORIC The generic name of a drug produced by numerous companies.

Generic Name: Paregoric

Dosage Form	Strength	Route
Liquid	Available in one strength only	Oral

When Prescribed: Paregoric is prescribed for the control of diarrhea and colic.

Precautions and Warnings: Paregoric is made from opium, which may be habit forming.

Side Effects and Adverse Reactions: Constipation, nausea, vomiting.

PAVABID® (Marion Laboratories)

Generic Name: Papaverine hydrochloride

Dosage Form	Strength	Route
Capsule (Time Release)	150 mg	Oral

When Prescribed: Pavabid is prescribed for use by patients with certain heart conditions and/or for the treatment of obstruction or spasm of blood vessels.

Precautions and Warnings: Should be used only under close supervision of a physician.

Side Effects and Adverse Reactions: Nausea, abdominal distress, loss of appetite, constipation, depression, drowsiness, sweating, headache, diarrhea, skin rash, loss of balance.

PEDIAMYCIN® (Ross Laboratories)

Generic Name: Erythromycin ethylsuccinate

Dosage Form	Strength	Route
Liquid	200 mg/5 ml	Oral
	400 mg/5 ml	Oral
Suspension	200 mg/5 ml	Oral
Drops	100 mg/dropper	Oral

When Prescribed: Pediamycin is the antibiotic erythromycin in pleasant-tasting forms which make it especially suitable for children. Pediamycin is prescribed for a wide variety of infections.

Precautions and Warnings: Pediamycin is an antibiotic which can cause an allergic reaction in susceptible individuals.

Side Effects and Adverse Reactions: Abdominal cramping, discomfort, nausea, vomiting and diarrhea. Other reactions include super-infection by nonsusceptible organisms, hives, rash and fainting.

PENICILLIN G POTASSIUM
400, 000 Units The generic name of a drug produced by numerous companies in various forms and strengths.
Also marketed as:
KESSO–PEN®, McKesson;
PENTIDS®, E. R. Squibb;
PFIZERPEN® G, Pfizer;
QIDPEN® G, Mallinckrodt.

Generic Name: Potassium penicillin G

Dosage Form	Strength	Route
Tablet	250 mg*	Oral

When Prescribed: Penicillin G potassium is prescribed for the treatment of mild to moderately severe infections by organisms which are susceptible to this type of penicillin. There are different types of penicillin, each of which is effective in different infections. Your physician has determined which type is the proper one to use in your particular case.

Precautions and Warnings: Serious hypersensitivity (allergic) reactions can occur in susceptible individuals. For maximum absorption, dosage should be given on an empty stomach. If any of the symptoms listed below occurs, consult your physician immediately.

Side Effects and Adverse Reactions: Nausea, vomiting, heartburn, diarrhea, black hairy tongue, skin rash, skin eruptions, hives, chills, fever, swelling, pain in the joints, fainting, swelling in the throat, anemia, sore mouth, super-infection by nonsusceptible organisms.

PENICILLIN V POTASSIUM

400,000 Units The generic name of a drug produced by numerous companies in various forms and strengths. Also marketed as:

PEN–VEE K®, Wyeth;
V–CILLIN K®, Eli Lilly Co.;
VEETIDS®, Squibb.

Generic Name: Penicillin V potassium

Dosage Form	Strength	Route
Tablet	250 mg*	Oral

When Prescribed: Penicillin V potassium is prescribed for the treatment of mild to moderately severe infections by organisms which are susceptible to this type of penicillin. There are different types of penicillin, each of which is effective in different infections. Your physician determines which type is the proper one to use in your particular case.

Precautions and Warnings: Serious hypersensitivity (allergic) reactions can occur in susceptible individuals. For maximum absorption, dosage should be given on an empty stomach. If any of the symptoms listed below occurs, consult your physician immediately.

Side Effects and Adverse Reactions: Nausea, vomiting, heartburn, diarrhea, changes in color/texture of oral membranes, skin rash, skin eruptions, hives, chills, fever, swelling, pain in joints, fainting, difficult breathing, anemia, sore mouth, super-infection by nonsusceptible organisms.

PENTIDS® (E. R. Squibb and Sons)

Generic Name: Potassium penicillin G

Dosage Form	Strength	Route
Syrup	200,000 units	Oral
	400,000 units*	Oral
Tablet	200,000 units	Oral
	400,000 units	Oral
	800,000 units	Oral

When Prescribed: See Penicillin G Potassium.

Precautions and Warnings: See Penicillin G Potassium.

Side Effects and Adverse Reactions: See Penicillin G Potassium.

PEN-VEE® K (Wyeth Laboratories)

Generic Name: Penicillin V potassium

Dosage Form	Strength	Route
Tablet	125 mg 200,000 units	Oral
	250 mg 400,000 units*	Oral
	500 mg 800,000 units	Oral
Liquid	125 mg 200,000 units	Oral
	250 mg 400,000 units	Oral

When Prescribed: See Penicillin V Potassium.

Precautions and Warnings: See Penicillin V Potassium.

Side Effects and Adverse Reactions: See Penicillin V Potassium.

PERCODAN® (Endo Laboratories, Inc.)

Generic Name: Oxycodone hydrochloride, oxycodone terephthalate, aspirin, phenacetin, caffeine

Dosage Form	Strength	Route
Tablet	Full strength*	Oral
Tablet (Perdocan demi)	Half strength	Oral

When Prescribed: Percodan is prescribed for the relief of moderate to moderately severe pain. Percodan contains a narcotic pain reliever and therefore is prescribed only when weaker medication is deemed ineffective.

Precautions and Warnings: Percodan can produce drug dependence and therefore has the potential for abuse. Physical and/or psychological dependence can occur. Patients using this drug should not drive or use dangerous machinery. Percodan should not be taken with alcohol, tranquilizers, sedatives or sleeping pills. This drug is not recommended for use during pregnancy nor for use by children.

Side Effects and Adverse Reactions: Light-headedness, dizziness, sedation, nausea, vomiting, altered states of mood, constipation and itching.

PERIACTIN® (Merck Sharp and Dohme)

Generic Name: Cyproheptadine hydrochloride

Dosage Form	Strength	Route
Tablet	4 mg*	Oral
Syrup	2 mg/5 ml	Oral

When Prescribed: Periactin is an antihistamine prescribed for nasal congestion, hay fever and allergies; for swollen eyes due to pollen and food allergies; for mild skin allergies manifested as rash or hives; for allergic reactions from blood transfusions; and for various other allergic reactions.

Precautions and Warnings: Patients using this drug should not drive or operate dangerous machinery. Alcohol, tranquilizers, sedatives and sleeping pills should not be used with this drug. Mothers should not nurse while taking this drug.

Side Effects and Adverse Reactions: Drowsiness, dry mouth, dizziness, jitteriness, faintness, dryness of the mucous membranes, headache, nausea, rash, swelling, agitation, confusion, hallucinations, difficulty urinating, fatigue, restlessness, tremors, irritability, tingling or numbness in hands, excessive prespiration, chills, insomnia euphoria, loss of appetite, vomiting, diarrhea, constipation, irregular heart beat, tightness of chest, wheezing, rash, hives, visual disturbances, menstrual irregularities.

PERITRATE® (Parke-Davis)

Generic Name: Pentaerythritol tetranitrate

Dosage Form	Strength	Route
Tablet	10 mg	Oral
	20 mg	Oral
	40 mg	Oral
Tablet S.A. (Time Release)	80 mg	Oral

When Prescribed: Peritrate is prescribed for patients with coronary artery disease (a form of heart disease) to reduce the frequency, intensity and duration of chest pain (angina pectoris). Peritrate is not intended to relieve the pain of the angina (in which case a drug containing nitroglycerin is often used) but to prevent the occurrence of such episodes.

Precautions and Warnings: Angina pectoris results from heart disease, which can be fatal. Close interaction with your physician is indicated for any heart condition. Your physician should be advised if any of the symptoms listed below appear.

Side Effects and Adverse Reactions: Rash, headache, gastrointestinal distress, flushing, dizziness, weakness, nausea, vomiting, restlessness, perspiration, fainting. Some side effects may be enhanced when this drug is used with alcohol.

PERSANTINE (Boehringer Ingelheim Ltd.)

Generic Name: Dipyridamole

Dosage Form	Strength	Route
Tablet	25 mg	Oral
	50 mg	Oral
	75 mg	Oral

When Prescribed: Persantine is prescribed for the long-term management of attacks of anginal pectoris which result from heart disease. Persantine is not to be used for the pain of an acute anginal attack but rather to help prevent such an attack. Acute angina attacks are usually treated with nitroglycerin. Persantine works by increasing the blood flow in coronary vessels of the heart.

Precautions and Warnings: Angina pectoris results from heart disease which could be fatal. Report any side effects or unusual reactions to your physician at once.

Side Effects and Adverse Reactions: Headache, nausea, flushing, weakness, fainting, gastrointestinal upset, rash, chest or shoulder pain.

PHENAPHEN® with CODEINE NO. 3 (A. H. Robins Company)

Generic Name: Codeine Phosphate, acetaminophen

Dosage Form	Strength	Route
Capsule	No. 2	Oral
	No. 3*	Oral
	No. 4	Oral

When Prescribed: Phenaphen is prescribed for the relief of pain.

Precautions and Warnings: This preparation may be habit forming with prolonged or overuse. If drowsiness occurs, you should not drive or operate machinery. Should not be taken with alcohol, tranquilizers, sedatives or sleeping pills. The safe use of Phenaphen with codeine during pregnancy has not been established.

Side Effects and Adverse Reactions: Drowsiness, nausea, constipation, lightheadedness, dizziness, euphoria, uneasiness, sedation, nausea and vomiting.

PHENERGAN® EXPECTORANT
(Wyeth Laboratories)

Generic Name: Promethazine, potassium guaiacolsulfonate, citric acid, sodium citrate, fluid extract ipecac, chloroform, alcohol

Dosage Form	Strength	Route
Liquid	Available in one strength only	Oral

When Prescribed: Phenergan Expectorant is prescribed for nasal and chest congestion due to hay fever, allergies or colds. This drug contains an expectorant which thins mucus, making it easier to pass from the respiratory tract. In addition, it contains vitamin C.

Precautions and Warnings: This drug contains a mild sedative. Patients using Phenergan should not drive or operate machinery. This drug should not be taken with alcohol, tranquilizers, sedatives or sleeping pills.

Side Effects and Adverse Reactions: Dryness of mouth, blurred vision, dizziness, changes in blood pressure, increased skin sensitivity to sunlight.

PHENERGAN® EXPECTORANT
with CODEINE (Wyeth Laboratories)

Generic Name: Promethazine, potassium guaiacolsulfonate, citric acid, sodium citrate, fluid extract ipecac, chloroform, alcohol, codeine

Dosage Form	Strength	Route
Liquid	Available in one strength only	Oral

When Prescribed: Phenergan Expectorant with Codeine is prescribed for the same reasons as Phenergan Expectorant. In addition, the former contains codeine, which will suppress the coughs that may accompany such conditions.

Precautions and Warnings: In addition to the precautions and warnings for Phenergan Expectorant, this drug may be habit forming.

Side Effects and Adverse Reactions: In addition to the side effects possible with Phenergan Expectorant, this drug may cause constipation or nausea.

PHENERGAN® VC EXPECTORANT
(Wyeth Laboratories)

Generic Name: Promethazine, potassium guaiacolsulfonate, citric acid, sodium citrate, phenylephrine hydrochloride, fluid extract ipecac, chloroform, alcohol

Dosage Form	Strength	Route
Liquid	Available in one strength only	Oral

When Prescribed: Phenergan VC Expectorant is prescribed for the same reasons as Phenergan Expectorant. In addition, it contains phenylephrine hydrochloride, which will help dry up mucous membranes.

Precautions and Warnings: See Phenergan Expectorant.

Side Effects and Adverse Reactions: See Phenergan Expectorant.

PHENERGAN® VC EXPECTORANT with CODEINE (Wyeth Laboratories)

Generic Name: Promethazine, potassium guaiacolsulfonate, citric acid, sodium citrate, phenylephrine hydrochloride, fluid extract ipecac, chloroform, alcohol, codeine

Dosage Form	Strength	Route
Liquid	Available in one strength only	Oral

When Prescribed: Phenergan VC Expectorant with Codeine is prescribed for nasal and chest congestion due to hay fever, allergies or colds. This drug contains an expectorant which thins mucous, an agent which will dry mucous membranes, and codeine which will help suppress coughs.

Precautions and Warnings: Codeine may be habit forming. If drowsiness occurs you should not drive or operate dangerous machinery. Phenergan VC Expectorant with Codeine should not be taken with alcohol, sleeping pills, sedatives, or tranquilizers.

Side Effects and Adverse Reactions: Dryness of mouth, blurred vision, dizziness, increased sensitivity to sunlight, constipation, nausea.

PHENOBARBITAL The generic name for a drug produced by numerous companies in various forms and strengths.

Generic Name: Phenobarbital

Dosage Form	Strength	Route
Tablet	15 mg	Oral
	30 mg*	Oral

When Prescribed: Phenobarbital is a sedative and sleep-inducing drug which is prescribed for a variety of reasons, among which are anxiety, tension, restlessness, hyperactivity, insomnia and epilepsy.

Precautions and Warnings: Phenobarbital may be habit forming. Patients taking this drug should not drive or operate machinery. Phenobarbital should not be taken with alcohol, sedatives, sleeping pills or tranquilizers. The safe use of phenobarbital in pregnancy has not been established.

Side Effects and Adverse Reactions: Drowsiness, hangover, dizziness, loss of balance, headache, nausea, skin eruptions, rash, hives, excitement, confusion, depression, lethargy, vomiting.

PLACIDYL® (Abbott Laboratories)

Generic Name: Ethchlorvynol

Dosage Form	Strength	Route
Capsule	100 mg	Oral
	200 mg	Oral
	500 mg	Oral
	750 mg	Oral

When Prescribed: Placidyl is used as a sleep-inducing agent for insomnia.

Precautions and Warnings: This drug should not be taken before driving or operating machinery. Placidyl should not be taken with alcohol, sedatives, tranquilizers or other sleeping pills. Physical and/or psychological dependency on this drug can be developed with overuse. Placidyl should not be taken during pregnancy. The safe use of this drug in nursing mothers has not been established.

Side Effects and Adverse Reactions: Low blood pressure, nausea, vomiting, upset stomach, aftertaste, blurring of vision, dizziness, facial numbness, hives, rash, hangover, anxiety, loss of balance, slurring of speech, memory loss, loss of appetite, fainting, weakness, prolonged sedation. Abrupt withdrawal may cause convulsions.

POLARAMINE® (Schering Corporation)

Generic Name: Dexchlorpheniramine maleate (alcohol in syrup and expectorant, dexchlorpheniramine maleate, isoephedrine sulfate), guaifenesin in expectorant)

Dosage Form	Strength	Route
Syrup	2 mg/5 ml	Oral
Expectorant	2 mg/5 ml	Oral
Tablets	2 mg	Oral
	4 mg	Oral
Repetabs® (Timed Release)	6 mg	Oral

When Prescribed: Polaramine is prescribed for the relief of symptoms from hay fever, nasal congestion, allergic skin rash, itching, poison ivy or oak, insect bites, drug reactions, asthma, and other disorders that are treatable with antihistamines. The expectorant is prescribed for the relief of the above when cough is a complicating factor.

Precautions and Warnings: If drowsiness occurs you should not drive or operate dangerous machinery.

Side Effects and Adverse Reactions: Drowsiness, dizziness, nausea, restlessness, dry mouth, weakness, loss of appetite, headache, nervousness, frequent urination, heartburn, double vision, sweating, urinary difficulties, skin irritation.

POLYCILLIN® (Bristol Laboratories)

Generic Name: Ampicillin

Dosage Form	Strength	Route
Capsule	250 mg*	Oral
	500 mg	Oral
Liquid	125 mg/5 ml	Oral
	250 mg/5 ml	Oral
	500 mg/5 ml	Oral
Pediatric drops	100 mg/5 ml	Oral

When Prescribed: Polycillin is a synthetic penicillin that is effective in a wide variety of infections.

Precautions and Warnings: Polycillin should not be taken by people who are allergic to penicillin. The use of any penicillin should be discontinued and your physician notified if any abnormal symptoms appear.

Side Effects and Adverse Reactions: Nausea, vomiting, chest or stomachache, diarrhea, blackening of tongue, skin rash, hives, chills, fever, swelling, pain in joints, fainting, super-infection by nonsusceptible organisms.

POLY-VI-FLOR® (Mead Johnson Laboratories)

Generic Name: Multiple vitamins plus fluoride

Dosage Form	Strength	Route
Tablet	Available in one strength only	Oral (chewable)
Drops	Available in one strength only	Oral

When Prescribed: This preparation is prescribed for children to prevent vitamin deficiencies and to supply fluoride for prevention of tooth decay in areas where the fluoride content of the water is low.

Precautions and Warnings: Poly-Vi-Flor should only be used in areas where the fluoride content of the drinking water is below 0.7 parts per million. Do not give more than prescribed. Keep out of reach of children.

Side Effects and Adverse Reactions: Overuse can lead to fluoride poisoning. Rash may develop in children allergic to this preparation.

POTASSIUM CHLORIDE: The generic name for a drug produced by numerous companies and marketed in various forms and strengths. Also marketed as:
K-LOR, Abbott;
K-LYTE/CL, Mead Johnson Pharmaceutical;
KAOCHLOR, Warren-Teed;
KAY CIEL, Berlex;
KEFF, Lemmon;
KLOR-CON, Upsher-Smith;
KLORVESS, Dorsey;
KOLYUM, Pennwalt;
RUM-K, Fleming;
SLOW-K, Ciba.

Generic Name: Potassium chloride

Dosage Form	Strength	Route

Available in various forms and strengths to be taken orally.

When Prescribed: Potassium chloride is prescribed to replace potassium, an essential salt, in patients who are deficient in potassium. Potassium deficiency can result from the use of drugs that control blood pressure, among other reasons.

Precautions and Warnings: Potassium-containing drugs are often upsetting to the stomach. For this reason many of the drugs will be in the form of a tablet or powder which should be dissolved completely before taking. Gastrointestinal upset can be reduced if the drug is taken with meals. If the drug is in a liquid form it should be sipped slowly over a five-to-ten-minute period.

Side Effects and Adverse Reactions: Nausea, vomiting, diarrhea, abdominal discomfort.

PREDNISONE
The generic name of a drug produced by numerous companies in various strengths. Also marketed as:
DELTASONE®, Upjohn;
DELTRA®, Merck Sharp and Dohme;
METICORTEN®, Schering.

Generic Name: Prednisone

Dosage Form	Strength	Route
Tablet	5.0 mg	Oral

When Prescribed: Prednisone is a hormone which is primarily noted for its potent anti-inflammatory effect. It is prescribed for endocrine disorders, arthritis, collagen disease, skin diseases, allergic reactions, eye diseases, respiratory diseases, blood disorders, cancer of the blood, water retention and various other diseases.

Precautions and Warnings: Prednisone is a potent drug which should be used only under close supervision of a physician. Patients should not receive smallpox immunization or other inoculations while on Prednisone therapy.

Side Effects and Adverse Reactions: Water retention, heart failure, muscle weakness, loss of muscle, bone fractures, ulcer, abdominal distention, wounds that heal slowly, thin fragile skin, skin eruptions, increased sweating, convulsions, dizziness, headache, menstrual irregularities, masculinization of females, suppression of growth in children, decreased ability to withstand stress, intensification of existing diabetes, cataracts, glaucoma.

PRELUDIN® ENDURETS® (Boehringer Ingelheim Ltd.)

Generic Name: Phenmetrazine hydrochloride

Dosage Form	Strength	Route
Enduret (prolonged-action tablet)	50 mg 75 mg*	Oral Oral

When Prescribed: Preludin Endurets are a prolonged-action tablet containing a drug which is used for weight reduction in overweight individuals who cannot lose sufficient weight by diet alone. Preludin Endurets act by decreasing the appetite. They are usually prescribed for a short period of time (a few weeks), during which time the diet is controlled.

Precautions and Warnings: Preludin is a stimulant which may impair judgment. Patients should use caution in driving or operating machinery. Preludin is related to amphetamines, which have potential for abuse resulting in physical and/or psychological dependence. The safe use of this drug in pregnancy has not been established.

Side Effects and Adverse Reactions: Rapid or irregular heart beat, high blood pressure, overstimulation, restlessness, dizziness, insomnia, changes in mood, tremor, headache, psychotic episodes, dryness of mouth, unpleasant taste, diarrhea, constipation, gastrointestinal pain, hives, impotence, changes in sex drive.

PREMARIN® (Ayerst Laboratories)

Generic Name: Conjugated estrogens

Dosage Form	Strength	Route
Tablet	0.3 mg	Oral
	0.625 mg	Oral
	1.25 mg*	Oral
	2.5 mg	Oral

Note: Also available in vaginal cream and topical cream.

When Prescribed: Estrogens are secreted by the ovary and are responsible for the development and maintenance of the female reproductive system. Premarin is often prescribed for estrogen replacement for deficiencies caused by menopause, and other conditions where ovarian output of estrogen is diminished. Premarin may be prescribed for abnormal uterine bleeding due to hormonal imbalance. It is prescribed for the prevention of breast enlargement after childbirth and sometimes in the treatment of breast cancers. In males, it may be used in the treatment of cancer of the prostate.

Precautions and Warnings: Premarin is not recommended for use during pregnancy. Premarin should be used only under close supervision by your physician. Increased instances of dangerous side effects including cancer and blood clots have been reported with estrogen compounds. Should not be used for "prolonged" periods of time.

Side Effects and Adverse Reactions: Nausea, vomiting, loss of appetite, abdominal cramps, bloating, bleeding or spotting at times other than menstruation, breast tenderness and enlargement, reduction in milk production when given after childbirth, in males

PRINCIPEN® (E. R. Squibb and Sons)

Generic Name: Ampicillin trihydrate

Dosage Form	Strength	Route
Capsule	250 mg	Oral
	500 mg	Oral
Liquid	125 mg/5 ml	Oral
	250 mg/5 ml*	Oral

When Prescribed: Principen is a synthetic penicillin that is effective in a wide variety of infections.

Precautions and Warnings: Principen should not be taken by people who are allergic to penicillin. The use of any penicillin should be discontinued and your physician notified if any abnormal symptoms appear.

Side Effects and Adverse Reactions: Nausea, vomiting, chest or stomach pains, diarrhea, changes in color/texture of oral membranes, skin rash, hives, chills, fever, swelling, pain in joints, fainting, super-infection by non-susceptible organisms.

Premarin (Continued)

loss of sex drive and development of breasts, water retention, aggravation of migraine headaches, headache, allergic rash, dizziness, abnormal weight changes, inability to wear contact lenses, beard growth in females, loss of hair.

PRO-BANTHINE® (Searle and Company)

Generic Name: Propantheline bromide

Dosage Form	Strength	Route
Tablet	7.5 mg	Oral
	15 mg*	Oral

When Prescribed: Pro-Banthine is prescribed for the treatment of peptic ulcer. It may act by inhibiting gastrointestinal movements and acid secretion. This drug may cause drowsiness. If drowsiness occurs you should not drive or operate dangerous machinery.

Precautions and Warnings: Overdosage with this drug can lead to depression or arrest of breathing. Take only as directed.

Side Effects and Adverse Reactions: Drying of salivary secretions, dilation of pupils, blurred vision, nervousness, drowsiness, dizziness, insomnia, headache, loss of sense of taste, nausea, vomiting, constipation, impotence, allergic skin reactions, difficulty in urinating, decreased sweating in hot environments.

PROLOID® (Parke-Davis)

Generic Name: Thyroglobulin

Dosage Form	Strength	Route
Tablet	32 mg	Oral
	65 mg	Oral
	100 mg	Oral
	130 mg	Oral
	200 mg	Oral

When Prescribed: Proloid is prescribed to replace thyroid hormone in conditions where the production of hormone is low. It is thyroid hormone extracted from animals.

Precautions and Warnings: Proloid therapy requires frequent check-ups with your physician.

Side Effects and Adverse Reactions: No side effects have been reported in individuals when proper dosage has been maintained and no complicating illnesses are present. Symptoms of "overdose" include menstrual irregularities, nervousness, irregular heart beat, chest pain, arm pain.

PRONESTYL® (E. R. Squibb and Sons)

Generic Name: Procainamide hydrochloride

Dosage Form	Strength	Route
Capsule	250 mg	Oral
	375 mg	Oral
	500 mg	Oral
Tablet	250 mg	Oral
	375 mg	Oral
	500 mg	Oral

When Prescribed: Pronestyl is prescribed for the treatment of heart disorders characterized by premature or irregular heart beat.

Precautions and Warnings: Pronestyl is a potent drug which can regulate your heart beat. It is important that you be checked frequently by your physician during Pronestyl therapy.

Side Effects and Adverse Reactions: Loss of appetite, nausea, hives, rash, itching, vomiting, fever, chills, abdominal pains, bitter taste, diarrhea, weakness, mental depression, giddiness, psychosis, hallucinations, soreness of mouth, throat, gums, lupus-like lesions resulting from prolonged use (butterfly rash on face).

PROPOXYPHENE HCL: The generic name for a drug produced in various strengths by different companies. Also marketed as:
DARVON, Lilly;
SK-65, Smith, Kline, and French.

Generic Name: Propoxyphene HCl

Dosage Form	Strength	Route
Capsule	32 mg	Oral
	65 mg	Oral

When Prescribed: Propoxyphene HCl is prescribed for the relief of mild to moderate pain of any nature.

Precautions and Warnings: Propoxyphene has the potential for abuse and dependency, and it should not be used in people with addictive personalities. This drug should not be taken with alcohol, tranquilizers, sedatives, sleeping pills, or other central nervous system depressants. The safe use of this drug during pregnancy has not been established. Propoxyphene HCl is not recommended for children. If drowsiness occurs you should not drive or operate dangerous machinery.

Side Effects and Adverse Reactions: Dizziness, sedation, nausea, vomiting, constipation, abdominal pain, skin rash, light-headedness, headache, weakness, euphoria, uneasiness, visual disturbances.

PROPOXYPHENE HCL COMPOUND:
The generic name of a drug produced in various strengths and forms by a number of different companies. Also marketed as:
DARVON COMPOUND, Lilly;
SK-65 APAP, Smith, Kline, and French;
S-PAINACET, Saron;
WYGESIC, Wyeth.

Generic Name: Propoxyphene hydrochloride, aspirin, phenacetin, caffeine

Dosage Form	Strength	Route
Capsule	32 mg	Oral
	65 mg	Oral

When Prescribed: Propoxyphene HCl Compound is prescribed for the relief of moderate pain of any nature.

Precautions and Warnings: This drug should not be taken before undertaking potentially dangerous tasks such as driving a car or operating dangerous machinery. Propoxyphene HCl Compound should not be taken with alcohol, sedatives, tranquilizers, or sleeping pills. This drug can produce drug dependence which can be psychological or physical. The safe use of this compound in pregnancy has not been established. Not recommended for use in children.

Side Effects and Adverse Reactions: Dizziness, tiredness, nausea, vomiting, constipation, abdominal pain, skin rash, light-headedness, headache, weakness, euphoria, uneasiness, visual disturbances.

PROVERA® (The Upjohn Company)

Generic Name: Medroxyprogesterone acetate

Dosage Form	Strength	Route
Tablet	2.5 mg	Oral
	10 mg*	Oral

When Prescribed: Provera is a form of progesterone which is prescribed for the induction of menstruation in women for whom menstruation is irregular or absent, and for women (who are not pregnant) suffering from uterine bleeding or painful menstruation.

Precautions and Warnings: The use of progesterone substances such as Provera can result in a number of adverse side effects or reactions, some of which can be fatal. If you notice any side effect while taking this drug consult your physician at once.

Side Effects and Adverse Reactions: Breast tenderness, abnormal milk production, adverse effects on child if taken during pregnancy, hives, rash, skin eruptions, increase in facial hair, blood clots, abnormal menstrual bleeding, water retention, weight change, yellowing of skin or eyes, itching, mental depression, increase in blood pressure, changes in sex drive, changes in appetite, headache, nervousness, dizziness, fatigue, backache, loss of scalp hair.

PYRIDIUM® (Parke-Davis)

Generic Name: Phenazopyridine hydrochloride

Dosage Form	Strength	Route
Tablet	100 mg*	Oral
	200 mg	Oral

When Prescribed: Pyridium is prescribed for the symptomatic relief of pain, burning, urgency, frequency and other discomforts accompanying urination. These symptoms may result from infection, trauma, surgery, examination procedures or other factors which cause irritation of the lower urinary tract.

Precautions and Warnings: The reddish-orange discoloration of the urine is due to the drug and is normal.

Side Effects and Adverse Reactions: Gastrointestinal disturbances.

QUIBRON® (Mead Johnson Laboratories)

Generic Name: Theophylline, guaifenesin

Dosage Form	Strength	Route
Capsule	Available in one strength only	Oral
Liquid	Available in one strength only	Oral

When Prescribed: Quibron is prescribed for the relief of chest tightness and difficulty in breathing associated with asthma, bronchitis, emphysema or other lung disorders.

Precautions and Warnings: Quibron may exert a stimulating effect on the nervous system. Large doses may cause convulsions. Do not exceed recommended dosage.

Side Effects and Adverse Reactions: Gastric discomfort, nausea, vomiting, excitement, convulsions, muscle twitching, headache, insomnia, restlessness, heart flutters, diarrhea, frequent urination, increase in breathing rate.

QUINIDINE SULFATE:
The generic name of a drug produced by numerous companies in various forms and strengths. Also marketed as:
QUINIDEX®, Robins;
QUINORA®, Key.

Generic Name: Quinidine sulfate

Dosage Form	Strength	Route
Capsule (Lilly)	200 mg	Oral
Tablet	200 mg	Oral

When Prescribed: Quinidine Sulfate is prescribed for treatment of various disorders of the heart beat.

Precautions and Warnings: Quinidine Sulfate is a potent drug and its use requires constant monitoring by your physician.

Side Effects and Adverse Reactions: Ringing in the ears, headache, nausea, disturbed vision, change in heart beat, vomiting, abdominal pain, diarrhea, fever, loss of balance, apprehension, excitement, confusion, delirium, fainting, difficulty in hearing, flushing and itching of skin, easy bruising.

REGROTON® (USV Laboratories Inc.)

Generic Name: Chlorthalidone, reserpine

Dosage Form	Strength	Route
Tablet	Available in one strength only	Oral

When Prescribed: Regroton is a combination of drugs prescribed for the control of high blood pressure. Your physician has prescribed Regroton because the fixed combination of drugs in this compound is correct for you.

Precautions and Warnings: Regroton is a potent drug which should be used only under close supervision by your physician.

Side Effects and Adverse Reactions: Loss of appetite, gastric irritation, nausea, vomiting, diarrhea, constipation, nasal congestion, muscle cramps, dizziness, weakness, headache, drowsiness, mental depression, skin rashes, hives, anemia, restlessness, visual defects, impotence, painful urination, increased sensitivity to sunlight, yellowing of skin, yellow appearance of objects, slowing of heart, itching, skin eruptions, loss of appetite, nasal stuffiness.

RESERPINE The generic name for a drug produced by numerous companies in various strengths. Also marketed as:
SERPASIL®, Ciba;
RAU–SED®, E. R. Squibb.

Generic Name: Reserpine

Dosage Form	Strength	Route
Tablet	0.1 mg	Oral
	0.25 mg*	Oral

When Prescribed: Reserpine is prescribed to control mild forms of high blood pressure. It may also be prescribed in certain mental disorders.

Precautions and Warnings: This drug can produce severe depression in susceptible individuals. Discontinue drug at first sign of despondency, loss of appetite, early morning insomnia, impotence or self deprecation. Patients should inform an anesthesiologist of current or prior use of Reserpine. The safe use of this drug in pregnancy has not been established.

Side Effects and Adverse Reactions: Oversecretion of stomach acid, nausea, vomiting, loss of appetite, diarrhea, chest pain, irregular heart beat, slowing of heartbeat, drowsiness, depression, nervousness, anxiety, nightmares, tremors, dullness of feeling, deafness, eye problems, nasal congestion, itching, rash, dryness of mouth, headache, dizziness, fainting, impotence, decreased sex drive, painful urination, muscular aches, weight gain, breast enlargement, lactation, development of breasts in males.

RITALIN® (Ciba Pharmaceutical Company)

Generic Name: Methylphenidate hydrochloride

Dosage Form	Strength	Route
Tablet	5 mg	Oral
	10 mg*	Oral
	20 mg	Oral

When Prescribed: This drug is prescribed for a syndrome called attention deficit disorder (previously known as minimal brain dysfunction in children), for narcolepsy, a disorder of the sleep mechanism in which uncontrolled or abnormal sleep occurs, and also to treat mild depression or senile behavior.

Precautions and Warnings: Chronically abusive use of this drug can lead to psychological dependence with varying degrees of abnormal behavior. The safe use of this drug in pregnancy has not been established.

Side Effects and Adverse Reactions: Nervousness, insomnia, skin rash, hives, fever, pain in joints, skin eruptions, loss of appetite, nausea, dizziness, blood pressure and pulse changes (both up and down), abdominal pain, weight loss, anemia, scalp hair loss, abnormal movements or tremors, headache, irregular heart beat.

ROBAXIN® (A. H. Robins Company)

Generic Name: Methocarbamol

Dosage Form	Strength	Route
Tablet	500 mg	Oral
	750 mg*	Oral

When Prescribed: Robaxin is prescribed for the relief of discomfort associated with muscle-skeletal disorders. The relaxation brought about by Robaxin is thought to be due to a general nervous system depression.

Precautions and Warnings: Robaxin is not recommended for use during pregnancy or for nursing mothers. Safety and effectiveness of Robaxin in children under the age of 12 has not been established. If drowsiness occurs you should not drive or operate dangerous machinery.

Side Effects and Adverse Reactions: Light-headedness, dizziness, drowsiness, nausea, rash, eye irritation, visual disturbances, nasal congestion, blurred vision, headache, fever.

ROBAXISAL® (A. H. Robins Company)

Generic Name: Methocarbamol, aspirin

Dosage Form	Strength	Route
Tablet	500 mg	Oral
	750 mg	Oral

When Prescribed: Robaxisal is prescribed for the relief of discomfort associated with muscle-skeletal disorders. In Robaxisal, the skeletal muscle relaxant action of Methocarbamol is combined with the analgesic effects of aspirin. Often prescribed for "whiplash," acute strains, sprains and arthritis.

Precautions and Warnings: Since dizziness and drowsiness can occur, patients using Robaxisal should not undertake potentially dangerous tasks such as driving or operating machinery. This drug is not recommended for use during pregnancy or for nursing mothers. Safety and effectiveness of Robaxisal in children under the age of 12 has not been established.

Side Effects and Adverse Reactions: Light-headedness, dizziness, drowsiness, mild nausea, itching, rash, nasal congestion, conjunctivitis, blurred vision, headache, fever, stomach upset, constipation, diarrhea, chest congestion.

ROBITET® (A. H. Robins Company)

Generic Name: Tetracycline Hydrochloride

Dosage Form	Strength	Route
Capsule	250 mg	Oral
	500 mg	Oral
Syrup	125 mg/5 ml	Oral

When Prescribed: Robitet is an effective antibiotic prescribed for many different types of infection. It is often used in place of penicillin in patients who are allergic to penicillin.

Precautions and Warnings: Robitet should not be taken by people overly sensitive to tetracycline. Should be taken one hour before or two hours after meals. Milk, other dairy products and antacids interfere with absorption. If any of the side effects listed below occur, consult your physician immediately. Not recommended for pregnant women, infants or children under the age of 8.

Side Effects and Adverse Reactions: Exaggerated sunburn, super-infection by nonsusceptible organisms, loss of appetite, nausea, vomiting, diarrhea, inflammation of the tongue, difficulty in swallowing, stomach pains, inflammation of the bowel and genital region, skin rash, hives, swelling, fainting.

SALUTENSIN® (Bristol Laboratories)

Generic Name: Hydroflumethiazide, Reserpine

Dosage Form	Strength	Route
Tablet	Available in one strength only	Oral

When Prescribed: Salutensin is a combination of drugs which reduce blood pressure and help the body to pass water. This drug is prescribed for the reduction of high blood pressure resulting from a variety of disorders. Salutensin may be prescribed along with other drugs to reduce high blood pressure.

Precautions and Warnings: This drug should not be taken by nursing mothers. This drug can lead to imbalances in certain salts. Any side effect or adverse reaction should be reported to your physician.

Side Effects and Adverse Reactions: Loss of appetite, stomach irritation, nausea, vomiting, cramps, diarrhea, constipation, dryness of mouth and thirst, weakness, lethargy, drowsiness, restlessness, muscle cramps, frequent urination, urinary problems, dizziness, loss of balance, tingling of skin, headache, yellow appearance of objects, rash, nightmares, nasal congestion, weight gain, blurred vision, itching, fainting, rash, impotence, change in sex drive, increased salivation, depression, nervousness, anxiety, chest pains, deafness.

SECONAL® SODIUM (Eli Lilly and Company)

Generic Name: Sodium secobarbital

Dosage Form	Strength	Route
Capsule (Pulvules®)	50 mg	Oral
	100 mg*	Oral

When Prescribed: Seconal is a short-acting sedative and sleeping pill with a very prompt onset of effect. For use at home it is usually prescribed as a sleeping pill.

Precautions and Warnings: Patients who have taken Seconal should not drive or operate machinery. This drug should not be taken with alcohol, sedatives, tranquilizers or sleeping pills. Seconal is habit forming if abused. Should not be used for longer than two weeks.

Side Effects and Adverse Reactions: Excitement, hangover, pain, allergic reactions, nausea, vomiting.

SELSUN® (Abbott Laboratories)

Generic Name: Selenium sulfide, detergent

Dosage Form	Strength	Route
Liquid (shampoo)	Available in one strength only	Apply to scalp

When Prescribed: Selsun is a shampoo prescribed for the treatment of common dandruff and flaking of scalp.

Precautions and Warnings: Oiliness of the hair may increase following use of the lotion. Yellow or orange discoloration of gray or white hair may occur but can usually be avoided by careful rinsing. Safe use on infants has not been established.

Side Effects and Adverse Reactions: Increased sensitivity of scalp or adjacent areas.

SEPTRA® (Burroughs Wellcome Company)

Generic Name: Trimethoprim, sulfamethoxazole

Dosage Form	Strength	Route
Tablet	Regular strength*	Oral
Tablet	Double strength	Oral
Liquid	Available in one strength only	Oral

When Prescribed: Septra is a combination of drugs prescribed for the treatment of certain types of urinary tract infections and for certain other types of bacterial infections.

Precautions and Warnings: Septra is not recommended during pregnancy or for nursing mothers. If any of the side effects or adverse reactions listed below appear, consult your physician.

Side Effects and Adverse Reactions: Rash, sore throat, stomach upset, nausea, vomiting, abdominal pains, diarrhea, yellowing of skin, headache, body aches, depression, convulsions, hallucinations, ringing in the ears, dizziness, loss of balance, insomnia, apathy, fatigue, weakness, nervousness, fever, chills, urinary difficulties.

SER-AP-ES® (Ciba Pharmaceutical Company)

Generic Name: Reserpine, hydralazine, hydrochloride, hydrochlorothiazide

Dosage Form	Strength	Route
Tablet	Available in one strength only	Oral

When Prescribed: Ser-ap-es is prescribed for the control of high blood pressure. This drug is prescribed only after your physician has determined that the fixed combination of drugs in this preparation is correct for you.

Precautions and Warnings: Ser-ap-es is a potent drug which should be used only under close supervision of your physician. The safe use of this drug in pregnancy has not been established.

Side Effects and Adverse Reactions: Oversecretion of stomach acid, nausea, vomiting, loss of appetite, diarrhea, chest pains, heart flutters, slowing of heart, drowsiness, depression, nervousness, anxiety, nightmares, tremors, dull sensations, deafness, eye disorders, nasal congestion, itching, rash, hives, skin eruptions, painful or difficult urination, muscle aches, weight gain, breast enlargement, lactation, breast development in males, increased heart rate, numbness or tingling of skin, yellow skin or eyes, hepatitis, constipation, yellow appearance of objects, increased sensitivity to sunlight, anemia, changes in blood pressure, fever, chills, diminished sex drive.

SERAX® (Wyeth Laboratories)

Generic Name: Oxazepam

Dosage Form	Strength	Route
Capsule	10 mg	Oral
	15 mg*	Oral
	30 mg	Oral
Tablet	15 mg	Oral

When Prescribed: Serax is prescribed for a wide variety of problems to provide relief from tension, anxiety and related symptoms. It is used in a wide variety of physical and/or emotional disorders, also in skeletal muscle spasm, and to treat symptoms of acute alcohol withdrawal. This product has been found to be particularly useful in older patients.

Precautions and Warnings: The use of Serax during pregnancy should almost always be avoided. Excessive use of this drug can cause a dependency. If drowsiness occurs, patients should not drive or operate dangerous machinery. Serax can lower tolerance to alcohol.

Side Effects and Adverse Reactions: Drowsiness, dizziness, loss of balance, headache, fainting, rashes, nausea, slurred speech, shaking, change in sex drive, anxiety, visual disturbances, nightmares, excitation and confusion, disorientation, fever, euphoria.

SINEQUAN® (Pfizer Laboratories Division)

Generic Name: Doxepin HCl

Dosage Form	Strength	Route
Capsule	10 mg	Oral
	25 mg*	Oral
	50 mg	Oral
	75 mg	Oral
	100 mg	Oral
	150 mg	Oral
Concentrated liquid	Available in one strength only	Oral

When Prescribed: Sinequan is prescribed for relief from anxiety, tension, depression, sleep disturbances, guilt, lack of energy, fear, apprehension and worry resulting from both physical and psychological disorders.

Precautions and Warnings: Sinequan may interact with other drugs. Be sure your physician is advised of all drugs you are taking. This drug is not recommended for children under the age of 12. If drowsiness occurs you should not drive or operate dangerous machinery. Tolerance to alcohol may be lowered.

Side Effects and Adverse Reactions: Dry mouth, blurred vision, constipation, urinary difficulties, drowsiness, confusion, disorientation, hallucinations, numbness, tingling of skin, dizziness, loss of balance, rash, nausea, vomiting, indigestion, taste disturbances, diarrhea, loss of appetite, altered sex drive, impotence, ringing in the ears, weight gain, sweating, chills, fatigue, weakness, headache, loss of hair, development of breasts in males, enlargement of breasts in females, rapid heartbeat, increased sensitivity to sunlight.

SINGLET® (Dow Pharmaceuticals)

Generic Name: Phenylephrine hydrochloride, chlorpheniramine maleate, acetaminophen

Dosage Form	Strength	Route
Tablet	Available in one strength only	Oral

When Prescribed: Singlet is prescribed to reduce congestion, secretions, pain and fever resulting from colds, hay fever, sinus problems, flu, and other conditions.

Precautions and Warnings: This drug may have dangerous interactions with other drugs you may be taking. Singlet is not recommended for use by nursing mothers. If drowsiness occurs do not drive or operate dangerous machinery. Not recommended for children under 12.

Side Effects and Adverse Reactions: Drowsiness, restlessness, dry mouth, dizziness, weakness, loss of appetite, nausea, headache, nervousness, urinary problems, heartburn, double vision, skin irritations, nausea, vomiting, anxiety, tenseness, tremors, loss of color, respiratory difficulties, sleeplessness, convulsions, heart flutters.

SLOW-K® (Ciba Pharmaceutical Company)

Generic Name: Potassium chloride

Dosage Form	Strength	Route
Tablet	600 mg	Oral

When Prescribed: Slow-K is a preparation formulated to provide a controlled rate of release of potassium chloride in patients whose level of potassium is low. It is often prescribed for patients who are taking certain cardiovascular or high blood pressure drugs (diuretics) that tend to deplete the body of potassium. Because Slow-K can cause ulcers and bleeding, other forms of potassium supplementation are usually prescribed. Slow-K is usually prescribed only in individuals who cannot or will not take these other forms of medication.

Precautions and Warnings: Frequent determinations of potassium levels are necessary while taking this preparation.

Side Effects and Adverse Reactions: Nausea, vomiting, abdominal discomfort, diarrhea, changes in heart beat, skin rash.

SOMA® COMPOUND (Wallace Laboratories)

Generic Name: Carisoprodol, phenacetin, caffeine

Dosage Form	Strength	Route
Tablet	Available in one strength only	Oral

When Prescribed: Soma Compound combines a muscle relaxant, a pain reliever and a stimulant. It is prescribed for the relief of pain and stiffness in muscles and joints resulting from injury or a chronic problem such as arthritis.

Precautions and Warnings: This drug may impair your mental and/or physical abilities. Patients using this drug should not drive or operate machinery. Soma Compound should not be taken with alcohol, sedatives, tranquilizers or sleeping pills. The safe use of Soma Compound in pregnancy has not been established. Not recommended for use by nursing mothers or for children under 5.

Side Effects and Adverse Reactions: Drowsiness, light-headedness, dizziness, itching, nervousness, flutters of the heart, weakness, loss of balance, agitation, euphoria, confusion, disorientation, gastrointestinal disturbances, insomnia, frequent urination, headache, fainting, skin rash, burning eyes.

SORBITRATE® (Stuart Pharmaceuticals)

Generic Name: Isosorbide dinitrate

Dosage Form	Strength	Route
Tablet	5 mg 10 mg	Oral (chewable)
Tablet	2.5 mg 5 mg	Sublingual (dissolve under tongue)
Tablet	5 mg 10 mg 20 mg	Oral Oral Oral

When Prescribed: Sorbitrate is prescribed to reduce the number and severity of attacks of chest pain (angina pectoris) resulting from coronary artery disease.

Precautions and Warnings: Angina pectoris results from heart disease which can be fatal. Close interaction with your physician is indicated for any heart condition. Use of alcohol with this drug may increase the occurrence of side effects and adverse reactions.

Side Effects and Adverse Reactions: Headache, flushing, dizziness, weakness, nausea, vomiting, restlessness, pallor, perspiration, collapse, rash.

STELAZINE® (Smith Kline and French Laboratories)

Generic Name: Trifluoperazine hydrochloride

Dosage Form	Strength	Route
Tablet	1 mg	Oral
	2 mg*	Oral
	5 mg	Oral
	10 mg	Oral

When Prescribed: Stelazine is a potent drug prescribed for the management of certain mental disorders or for the control of the excessive anxiety, tension and agitation seen with emotional or physical disorders.

Precautions and Warnings: Stelazine may impair mental and/or physical abilities, especially during the first few days of therapy. Patients using this drug should not drive or operate machinery. Should not be taken with sedatives, alcohol, tranquilizers or sleeping pills.

Side Effects and Adverse Reactions: Drowsiness, dizziness, skin reactions, rash, dry mouth, insomnia, absence of menstruation, fatigue, muscular weakness, loss of appetite, lactation, blurred vision, tremors, jerky movements, muscle spasms, difficulty swallowing, abnormal facial expressions or movements, anemia, yellowing of skin or eyes, sexual disorders, skin eruptions, eye problems, increased severity of angina in some patients.

SUDAFED® (Burroughs Wellcome Company)

Generic Name: Pseudoephedrine hydrochloride

Dosage Form	Strength	Route
Syrup	30 mg/5 cc (Available without prescription)	Oral
Tablet	30 mg (Available without prescription)	Oral
	60 mg* (Must have prescription)	Oral

When Prescribed: Sudafed 60 mg is prescribed for relief of congestion of nose and/or ears resulting from colds, allergies, or other disorders.

Precautions and Warnings: Consult your physician if any of the side effects listed below occur. Use only if directed by physician if high blood pressure, heart disease, urinary retention, glaucoma or thyroid disease are present.

Side Effects and Adverse Reactions: Nervousness, dizziness, sleeplessness, nausea, headache.

SULTRIN (Ortho Pharmaceutical Corp.)

Generic Name: Sulfathiazole, Sulfa-
cetamide, Sulfabenzamide

Dosage Form	Strength	Route
Cream	Available in one strength only	Intravaginal
Vaginal tablet	Available in one strength only	Intravaginal

When Prescribed: Sultrin is prescribed for the treatment of vaginal infections. It may also be prescribed to treat vaginal odor that results from radiation therapy.

Precautions and Warnings: If relief is not obtained in six to ten days consult your physician again.

Side Effects and Adverse Reactions: This drug is well tolerated.

SUMYCIN® (E. R. Squibb and Sons)

Generic Name: Tetracycline hydrochloride

Dosage Form	Strength	Route
Capsule	250 mg*	Oral
	500 mg	Oral
Tablet	250 mg	Oral
	500 mg	Oral
Syrup	125 mg/5 cc	Oral

When Prescribed: Sumycin is an effective antibiotic prescribed for many different types of infection. It is often used in place of penicillin in patients who are allergic to penicillin.

Precautions and Warnings: Sumycin should not be taken by people overly sensitive to tetracycline. If any of the side effects listed below occur, consult your physician immediately. Not recommended for pregnant women, infants or children under the age of 8.

Side Effects and Adverse Reactions: Exaggerated sunburn, super-infection by nonsusceptible organisms, loss of appetite, nausea, vomiting, diarrhea, inflammation of the tongue, difficulty swallowing, stomach pains, inflammation of the bowel and genital region, skin rash, hives, swelling, fainting.

SYNALAR® (Syntex Laboratories, Inc.)

Generic Name: Fluocinolone acetonide

Dosage Form	Strength	Route
Cream	0.01 % 0.025%*	Topical (applied directly to affected area)
Ointment	0.025%	Topical (applied directly to affected area)
Solution	0.01 %	Topical (applied directly to affected area)

When Prescribed: Synalar is a synthetic form of a hormone normally produced in your body. It is prescribed to reduce inflammation and swelling in certain skin disorders.

Precautions and Warnings: Synalar is applied locally and is well tolerated. However, if any irritation develops consult your physician. Synalar is not for use in the eye. This drug should not be used for prolonged periods of time or in large amounts by pregnant women.

Side Effects and Adverse Reactions: Burning, itching, irritation, dryness, infected hair follicles, acne, loss of pigment, excessive hair growth, skin destruction.

SYNALGOS–DC® (Ives Laboratories, Inc.)

Generic Name: Dihydrocodeine bitartrate, promethazine hydrochloride, aspirin, phenacetin, caffeine

Dosage Form	Strength	Route
Capsule	Available in one strength only	Oral

When Prescribed: Synalgos–DC is prescribed for the relief of moderate to moderately severe pain in situations where your physician wishes to add a mild sedative effect. This preparation contains a narcotic similar to codeine in addition to a mild sedative, and weaker pain relievers.

Precautions and Warnings: Because it contains a substance similar to codeine, Synalgos–DC may be habit forming. If drowsiness occurs you should not drive or operate dangerous machinery. The safe use of this drug in pregnant patients has not been established. This drug is not recommended for children.

Side Effects and Adverse Reactions: Light-headedness, dizziness, drowsiness, sedation, nausea, vomiting, constipation, itching, skin reactions.

SYNTHROID® (Flint Laboratories)

Generic Name: Sodium levothyroxine

Dosage Form	Strength	Route
Tablet	.025 mg	Oral
	.050 mg	Oral
	.1 mg*	Oral
	.15 mg	Oral
	.2 mg	Oral
	.3 mg	Oral

When Prescribed: Synthroid is synthetically produced thyroid gland hormone. Synthroid is prescribed when the body produces insufficient thyroid hormone. This can be due to a variety of reasons, some of which are surgery, disease, birth defect and radiation.

Precautions and Warnings: Synthroid therapy should be closely regulated by your physician.

Side Effects and Adverse Reactions: There have been no side effects or adverse reactions reported in individuals where proper dosage has been maintained and no complicating illnesses are present.

TABLOID® BRAND A.P.C with CODEINE (Burroughs Wellcome Company)

Generic Name: Aspirin, phenacetin, caffeine, codeine phosphate

Dosage Form	Strength	Route
Tablet	No. 2—15 mg	Oral
	No. 3—30 mg	Oral
	No. 4—60 mg	Oral

When Prescribed: Tabloid A.P.C with codeine is prescribed for the relief of mild, moderate, and moderate to severe pain.

Precautions and Warnings: Codeine may be habit forming. If drowsiness occurs, you should not operate motor vehicles or dangerous machinery.

Side Effects and Adverse Reactions: Light-headedness, dizziness, sedation, nausea, vomiting, mood changes, constipation, itching, headache, ringing in ears, confusion, drowsiness, sweating, thirst, stomach irritation.

TAGAMET (Smith, Kline and French Laboratories)

Generic Name: Cimetidine

Dosage Form	Strength	Route
Tablet	300 mg	Oral

When Prescribed: Tagamet is prescribed for the treatment of duodenal ulcers and certain other disorders characterized by an increase in acid secretion in the stomach. It acts by reducing acid secretion in the stomach.

Precautions and Warnings: Tagamet is recommended only for the short term (up to eight weeks) treatment of ulcer. Nursing mothers should not take this drug.

Side Effects and Adverse Reactions: Diarrhea, muscular pain, dizziness, rash, enlargement of breasts in males, development of breasts in male, confusion.

TALWIN® (Winthrop Laboratories)

Generic Name: Pentazocine hydrochloride

Dosage Form	Strength	Route
Tablet	50 mg	Oral

When Prescribed: Talwin is a potent analgesic prescribed for the relief of moderate pain when less potent drugs are deemed ineffective.

Precautions and Warnings: Patients using this drug should not drive or operate dangerous machinery. Talwin can be habit forming if overused. Chronic prolonged use of this drug can produce adverse withdrawal symptoms. The safe use of this drug in pregnancy has not been established. Talwin should not be taken by children under 12.

Side Effects and Adverse Reactions: Nausea, vomiting, constipation, abdominal distress, loss of appetite, diarrhea, dizziness, light-headedness, sedation, euphoria, headache, weakness, disturbed dreams, insomnia, fainting, blurred vision, difficulty focusing, hallucinations, tremor, irritability, excitement, ringing in the ears, sweating, flushing, chills, rash, hives, puffiness of face, decrease in blood pressure, rapid heartbeat, difficulty urinating.

TANDEARIL® (Geigy Pharmaceuticals)

Generic Name: Oxyphenbutazone

Dosage Form	Strength	Route
Tablet	100 mg	Oral

When Prescribed: Tandearil is a potent drug prescribed for the relief of pain and inflammation of gout, various forms of arthritis and other painful joint disorders.

Precautions and Warnings: Tandearil is not a simple pain reliever and is never prescribed casually. Patients using this drug should undergo frequent physicals and tests. Adverse reactions can occur rapidly; therefore the patient should immediately report anything abnormal to his physician. Patients using this drug should not drive or operate machinery.

Side Effects and Adverse Reactions: Fever, sore throat, sores in the mouth, indigestion, heartburn, slow healing of cuts, blood which does not clot, easy bruising, dark or bloody stools, significant weight gain, water retention with swelling, stomach or intestinal cramps or pain, nausea, vomiting, diarrhea, bloating, swollen glands, hepatitis, purple spots on skin, itching, general skin eruptions, hives, pains in joints, fever, rash, blood in the urine, frequent urination, lack of urination, kidney stones, painful urination, high blood pressure, pain in the eyes, blurred vision, loss of hearing, increase in size of thyroid (in neck), general agitation, confusion, lethargy.

TEDRAL® (Parke-Davis)

Generic Name: Theophylline, ephedrine hydrochloride, phenobarbital (alcohol in elixir), guaifenesin in expectorant

Dosage Form	Strength	Route
Tablet (available without a prescription)	Available in one strength only	Oral
SA tablet (Time Release)	Available in one strength only	Oral
Liquid (expectorant)	Available in one strength only	Oral
Liquid (suspension)	Available in one strength only	Oral
Liquid (elixir)	Available in one strength only	Oral

When Prescribed: Tedral is prescribed for the relief of symptoms of bronchial asthma, asthmatic bronchitis, and other disorders where bronchial spasms cause difficulty in breathing.

Precautions and Warnings: The phenobarbital in Tedral may be habit forming. If drowsiness occurs you should not drive or operate dangerous machinery.

Side Effects and Adverse Reactions: Stomach or chest pains, irregular heart beat, nervousness, insomnia, difficulty in urinating, stimulation, drowsiness.

TELDRIN® (Menley and James Laboratories)

Generic Name: Chlorpheniramine maleate

Dosage Form	Strength	Route
Capsule	8 mg	Oral
	12 mg*	Oral

When Prescribed: Teldrin is an antihistamine recommended for the relief of symptoms of nasal congestion due to hay fever or allergy, allergic eye reactions (swelling), skin allergies, and for other allergic reactions.

Precautions and Warnings: If drowsiness occurs while taking this drug patients should not drive or operate machinery. Avoid alcoholic beverages while taking this product. Teldrin may cause excitability especially in children.

Side Effects and Adverse Reactions: Drowsiness, dizziness, dryness of mouth, gastrointestinal upset, increased heart rate.

Note: This drug is available without a prescription.

TENUATE® DOSPAN® (Merrell-National Laboratories)

Generic Name: Diethylpropion hydrochloride

Dosage Form	Strength	Route
Tablet	25 mg	Oral
Dospan® tablet (Time Release)	75 mg*	Oral

When Prescribed: Tenuate Dospan is a prolonged-action tablet containing a drug which is used for weight reduction in overweight individuals who cannot lose sufficient weight by diet alone. It is usually prescribed for a short period of time (a few weeks), during which time diet is controlled.

Precautions and Warnings: Tenuate is a stimulant which may impair judgment. Patients should use caution in driving or operating machinery. Tenuate is related to amphetamines, which have a potential for abuse resulting in physical and/or psychological dependence. Tenuate should not be taken by children under 12.

Side Effects and Adverse Reactions: Irregular heart beat, high blood pressure, overstimulation, restlessness, dizziness, insomnia, changes in mood, tremor, headache, psychotic episodes, dryness of mouth, unpleasant taste, diarrhea, constipation, gastrointestinal pain, hives, impotence, changes in sex drive, drowsiness, nervousness, anxiety, nausea, vomiting, diarrhea, constipation, rash, development of breasts in males, enlargement of breasts, menstrual difficulties, breathing difficulties, hair loss, muscle pain, urinary difficulties, increased sweating.

TERRAMYCIN® (Pfizer Laboratories Division)

Generic Name: Oxytetracycline hydrochloride, glucosamine hydrochloride

Dosage Form	Strength	Route
Capsule	125 mg	Oral
	250 mg*	Oral
Liquid	125 mg/5 ml	Oral

When Prescribed: Terramycin is an effective antibiotic prescribed for many different types of infection. It is often used in place of penicillin in patients who are allergic to penicillin.

Precautions and Warnings: Terramycin should not be taken by people overly sensitive to tetracycline. If any of the side effects listed below occur, consult your physician immediately. Not recommended for pregnant women, infants or children under the age of 8.

Side Effects and Adverse Reactions: Exaggerated sunburn, super-infection by nonsusceptible organisms, loss of appetite, nausea, vomiting, diarrhea, inflammation of the tongue, difficulty swallowing, stomach pains, inflammation of the bowel and genital region, skin rash, hives, swelling, fainting.

TETRACYCLINE
The generic name for a drug produced by numerous companies in various forms and strengths. Also marketed as:
ACHROMYCIN®, Lederle;
KESSO-TETRA®, McKesson;
ROBITET® SYRUP, Robins;
SK–TETRACYCLINE® SYRUP, Smith Kline and French;
SUMYCIN® SYRUP, Squibb;
TETRACYCLINE CAPSULES AND SYRUP, Rexall;
TETRACYN® CAPSULES/SYRUP, Pfizer.

Generic Name: Tetracycline hydrochloride

Dosage Form	Strength	Route
Capsule	250 mg*	Oral

When Prescribed: Tetracycline is an effective antibiotic prescribed for many different types of infection. It is often used in place of penicillin in patients who are allergic to penicillin.

Precautions and Warnings: Tetracycline should not be taken by people overly sensitive to this drug. If any of the side effects listed below occur, consult your physician immediately. Not recommended for pregnant women, infants or children under the age of 8.

Side Effects and Adverse Reactions: Exaggerated sunburn, super-infection by nonsusceptible organisms, loss of appetite, nausea, vomiting, diarrhea, inflammation of the tongue, difficulty swallowing, stomach pains, inflammation of the bowel and genital region, skin rash, hives, swelling, fainting.

TETRACYN® (Pfipharmecs Division of Pfizer Inc.)

Generic Name: Tetracycline hydrochloride

Dosage Form	Strength	Route
Capsule	250 mg	Oral
	500 mg	Oral
Liquid	125 mg/5 ml	Oral

When Prescribed: Tetracyn is an effective antibiotic prescribed for many different types of infection. It is often used in place of penicillin in patients who are allergic to penicillin.

Precautions and Warnings: Tetracyn should not be taken by people overly sensitive to tetracycline. Should be taken one hour before or two hours after meals. Food, milk, other dairy products and antacids interfere with absorption. If any of the side effects listed below occur, consult your physician immediately. Not recommended for pregnant women, infants or children under the age of 8.

Side Effects and Adverse Reactions: Exaggerated sunburn, super-infection by nonsusceptible organisms, loss of appetite, nausea, vomiting, diarrhea, inflammation of the tongue, difficulty swallowing, stomach pains, inflammation of the bowel and genital region, skin rash, hives, swelling, fainting.

TETREX® (Bristol Laboratories)

Generic Name: Tetracycline phosphate complex

Dosage Form	Strength	Route
Capsule	250 mg	Oral
	500 mg	Oral

When Prescribed: Tetrex is an effective antibiotic prescribed for many different types of infection. It is often used in place of penicillin in patients who are allergic to penicillin.

Precautions and Warnings: Tetrex should not be taken by people overly sensitive to tetracycline. If any of the side effects listed below occur, consult your physician immediately. Not recommended for pregnant women, infants or children under the age of 8.

Side Effects and Adverse Reactions: Exaggerated sunburn, super-infection by nonsusceptible organisms, loss of appetite, nausea, vomiting, diarrhea, inflammation of the tongue, difficulty swallowing, stomach pains, inflammation of the bowel and genital region, skin rash, hives, swelling, fainting.

THORAZINE® (Smith Kline and French Laboratories)

Generic Name: Chlorpromazine

Dosage Form	Strength	Route
Tablet	10 mg	Oral
	25 mg*	Oral
	50 mg	Oral
	100 mg	Oral
	200 mg	Oral
Capsule	30 mg	Oral
(Time	75 mg	Oral
Release)		
(Spansules®)	150 mg	Oral
	200 mg	Oral
	300 mg	Oral
Liquid	10 mg/5 ml	Oral
Suppository	25 mg	Rectal
	100 mg	Rectal

When Prescribed: Thorazine is a sedative prescribed for the management of certain types of mental illness, for the control of nausea and vomiting, for chronic hiccups, to control overactive children and in other instances where a reduction of anxiety or apprehension is desirable.

Precautions and Warnings: This drug may impair mental/and or physical abilities. Patients taking Thorazine should not drive or operate machinery. This drug should not be used with alcohol, tranquilizers, sleeping pills or sedatives. The safe use of this drug in pregnancy has not been established.

Side Effects and Adverse Reactions: Drowsiness, yellow skin or eyes, anemia, sore throat, low blood pressure, fainting, tremors, abnormal movements, abnormal facial movements or expression, skin eruptions, hives, breast enlargement, lactation, false positive pregnancy tests, lack of

THYROID TABLETS
The generic name for a drug produced by numerous companies in various strengths. Among them: Armour, Smith Kline and French, Warner-Chilcott, Fleming, Flint.

Generic Name: Thyroid hormone

Dosage Form	Strength	Route
Tablet	60 mg*	Oral

When Prescribed: Thyroid Tablets supply thyroid hormone either from natural or synthetic sources. Thyroid Tablets are prescribed when the body produces insufficient thyroid hormone. This can be due to a variety of reasons, some of which are surgery, disease, birth defect and radiation.

Precautions and Warnings: Thyroid therapy should be closely regulated by your physician.

Side Effects and Adverse Reactions: There have been no side effects or adverse reactions reported in individuals where proper dosage has been maintained and no complicating illnesses are present. Overdosage can result in irregular heartbeat, increased heart rate, weight loss, chest pains, tremors, headache, diarrhea, nervousness, insomnia, sweating, intolerance to heat and fever.

Thorazine (Continued)

menstruation, breast growth in males, dry mouth, nasal congestion, constipation, inability to urinate, dilation of pupils, jaundice, changes in eyes, fever.

TIGAN® (Beecham Laboratories)

Generic Name: Trimethobenzamide hydrochloride

Dosage Form	Strength	Route
Suppository (Pediatric)	100 mg	Rectal
Suppository	200 mg*	Rectal
Capsule	100 mg	Oral
	250 mg	Oral

When Prescribed: Tigan is prescribed for the control of nausea and vomiting. The suppository is particularly effective for frequent or prolonged vomiting where the oral dose may be regurgitated.

Precautions and Warnings: Since drowsiness may occur, patients should not drive or operate machinery. The safe use of Tigan in pregnancy has not been established.

Side Effects and Adverse Reactions: Tremors, jerky movements, blurring of vision, coma, convulsion, depression of mood, diarrhea, disorientation, dizziness, drowsiness, headache, yellow skin or eyes, muscle cramps, allergic skin reactions.

TIMOPTIC (Merck, Sharp and Dohme)

Generic Name: Timolol maleate

Dosage Form	Strength	Route
Solution (Eye drop)	0.25%	Eyedrop
	0.50%	Eyedrop

When Prescribed: Timoptic is prescribed to lower elevated pressure in the eye that results from various disorders including glaucoma.

Precautions and Warnings: This drug is not recommended for use in children.

Side Effects and Adverse Reactions: Eye irritation, rash, reduction of heart rate.

TOFRANIL® (Geigy Pharmaceuticals)

Generic Name: Imipramine hydrochloride

Dosage Form	Strength	Route
Tablet	10 mg	Oral
	25 mg*	Oral
	50 mg	Oral

When Prescribed: Tofranil is prescribed for the relief of symptoms of depression. It may also be prescribed to control daytime frequency of urination and to control bed-wetting in individuals older than 6.

Precautions and Warnings: This drug can impair mental and/or physical abilities. Alcohol should not be used with this drug. Tofranil can lead to serious and sometimes fatal reactions if taken with certain other drugs. Be sure to inform your physician of all drugs you take. Mothers should not nurse while taking this drug.

Side Effects and Adverse Reactions: Changes in blood pressure, irregular heart beat, stroke, fainting, confusion, hallucinations, disorientation, delusions, anxiety, restlessness, agitation, insomnia, nightmares, numbness or tingling sensation, incoordination, loss of balance, tremors, ringing in the ears, dry mouth, blurred vision, trouble adapting to changing light, dilation of pupils, constipation, difficulty urinating, allergic skin disorders, anemia, sore throat, nausea, vomiting, heartburn, strange taste, abdominal cramps, black tongue, breast enlargement in males, breast enlargement and lactation in females, change in sexual behavior, swelling of testicles, yellow skin or eyes, change in weight, perspi-

TOLECTIN (McNeil Laboratories)

Generic Name: Tolmetin Sodium

Dosage Form	Strength	Route
Capsule	400 mg	Oral
Tablet	200 mg	Oral

When Prescribed: Tolectin is prescribed for the relief of pain and inflammation of arthritis. It is as effective as aspirin in reducing pain and inflammation but is usually better tolerated in the stomach.

Precautions and Warnings: This drug is not recommended for pregnant women or nursing mothers.

Side Effects and Adverse Reactions: Nausea, indigestion, abdominal pain, gastrointestinal distress, gas, diarrhea, constipation, vomiting, stomach upset, headache, weakness, chest pain, fainting, swelling, dizziness, light-headedness, nervousness, drowsiness, insomnia, depression, skin rash, itching, skin irritation, ringing in the ears.

TOFRANIL (Continued)

ration, frequent urination, dizziness, weakness, fatigue, loss of appetite, diarrhea, black tongue, loss of hair.

TOLINASE® (The Upjohn Company)

Generic Name: Tolazamide

Dosage Form	Strength	Route
Tablet	100 mg	Oral
	250 mg	Oral
	500 mg	Oral

When Prescribed: Tolinase is prescribed to lower blood sugar when blood sugar is high due to mild to moderately severe adult onset diabetes. It acts by helping to release the body's own insulin.

Precautions and Warnings: Patients taking Tolinase must be under continuous medical supervision. Your physician will ask you to check your urine daily for sugar. This drug does not replace the need to restrict diet. This drug is not recommended for use by the pregnant diabetic patient.

Side Effects and Adverse Reactions: Nausea, vomiting, gas, itching, rash, weakness, fatigue, loss of balance, dizziness, depression, headache, skin sensitivity to sunlight following ingestion of alcohol.

TRANXENE® (Abbott Laboratories)

Generic Name: Clorazepate dipotassium

Dosage Form	Strength	Route
Capsule	3.75 mg	Oral
	7.5 mg*	Oral
	15.0 mg	Oral
Tablet	22.5 mg	Oral
	11.25 mg	Oral

When Prescribed: Tranxene is prescribed for the relief of anxiety resulting from neurotic conditions as well as anxiety which can accompany diseases.

Precautions and Warnings: Patients taking this drug should not drive or operate machinery. Tranxene should not be taken with alcohol, sedatives, tranquilizers, or sleeping pills. A physical and/or psychological dependence on Tranxene can occur. This drug is not recommended for pregnant women or nursing mothers and is not recommended for use in patients under the age of 18.

Side Effects and Adverse Reactions: Drowsiness, dizziness, gastrointestinal complaints, nervousness, blurred vision, dry mouth, headache, mental confusion, insomnia, rash, fatigue, loss of balance, urinary difficulties, irritability, double vision, depression, slurred speech.

TRIAVIL® (Merck Sharp and Dohme)

Generic Name: Perphenazine, amitriptyline hydrochloride

Dosage Form	Strength	Route
Tablet	2–25*	Oral
	4–25	Oral
	2–10	Oral
	4–10	Oral

When Prescribed: Triavil is prescribed for various psychological problems characterized by anxiety and depression. This drug is used to control a wide variety of mental disorders.

Precautions and Warnings: Patients using this drug should not drive or operate machinery. Triavil should not be taken with alcohol, sedatives, sleeping pills or tranquilizers. This drug is not recommended for use in pregnant patients, nursing mothers, or in children.

Side Effects and Adverse Reactions: Tremors, jerky movements, skin eruptions, hives, rash, increased sensitivity to sunlight, asthma, fainting, swelling, lactation, breast enlargement (male and female), menstrual disturbances, excitement, changes in blood pressure, rapid heartbeat, dry mouth, salivation, headache, loss of appetite, nausea, vomiting, constipation, urinary frequency, blurred vision, nasal congestion, increased appetite, convulsions, change of skin color, impotence, yellow skin or eyes, eye disorders, nightmares, numbness or tingling, insomnia, loss of balance, ringing in ears, fatigue, dizziness, drowsiness, abnormal, uncontrollable movements of tongue or face, black tongue, loss of appetite, increased perspiration, loss of hair.

TRI-VI-FLOR® (Mead Johnson Nutritional Division)

Generic Name: Vitamins A, D, C, Fluoride

Dosage Form	Strength	Route
Liquid	Available in one strength only	Oral
Tablet	Available in one strength only	Oral

When Prescribed: Tri-Vi-Flor is prescribed for infants and children to prevent vitamin deficiencies and to supply fluoride for the prevention of tooth decay in areas where the fluoride content of the water is low.

Precautions and Warnings: Tri-Vi-Flor should only be used in areas where the fluoride content of the drinking water is below 0.7 parts per million. Do not give more than prescribed. Keep out of reach of children.

Side Effects and Adverse Reactions: Overuse can lead to fluoride poisoning. Rash may develop in children allergic to this preparation.

TUINAL® (Eli Lilly and Company)

Generic Name: Sodium secobarbital, sodium amobarbital

Dosage Form	Strength	Route
Capsule (Pulvules®)	50 mg	Oral
	100 mg	Oral
	200 mg*	Oral

When Prescribed: Tuinal is a rapidly-acting, long-duration combination of drugs (barbiturates) prescribed to induce sleep in individuals with insomnia.

Precautions and Warnings: This drug is a barbiturate which may be habit forming. Patients who have taken this drug should not drive or operate machinery. Tuinal should not be combined with alcohol, tranquilizers, sedatives or sleeping pills. Do not withdraw abruptly.

Side Effects and Adverse Reactions: Excitement, hangover, pain, allergic reactions, drowsiness, lethargy.

TUSS-ORNADE® (Smith Kline and French Laboratories)

Generic Name: Caramiphen edisylate, chlorpheniramine maleate, phenylpropanolamine hydrochloride, isopropamide iodide

Dosage Form	Strength	Route
Capsule (Spansules®)	Available in one strength only	Oral
Liquid (contains alcohol)	Available in one strength only	Oral

When Prescribed: Tuss-Ornade is prescribed for relief from coughing, upper respiratory congestion, and "runny nose" associated with the common cold, sinus infections, and allergies.

Precautions and Warnings: Tuss-Ornade should not be taken with certain drugs prescribed for high blood pressure. If drowsiness or blurred vision occurs you should not operate a car or machinery or participate in activities where alertness is required.

Side Effects and Adverse Reactions: Nausea, vomiting, dry mouth, nervousness, dizziness, headache, drowsiness, visual disturbances, mental confusion, painful urination, skin disorders, diarrhea, rash, chest pain, heart flutters, tremors, convulsions, dryness of nose, insomnia, abdominal pain, loss of coordination, loss of appetite, constipation.

TYLENOL® with CODEINE (McNeil Laboratories, Inc.)

Generic Name: Acetaminophen, codeine

Dosage Form	Strength	Route
Tablet	No 1	Oral
	No 2	Oral
	No 3*	Oral
	No 4	Oral
Elixir (contains alcohol)	Available in one strength only	Oral

When Prescribed: Tylenol with codeine is prescribed for the relief of pain of various causes, and for the relief of aches, pain, and coughing that may be symptoms of colds or flu.

Precautions and Warnings: Tylenol with codeine contains a narcotic pain reliever which may be habit forming. This preparation may cause drowsiness, therefore driving motor vehicles or operating dangerous machinery is discouraged while taking this treatment.

Side Effects and Adverse Reactions: Drowsiness, constipation, nausea, light headedness, dizziness, vomiting, mood changes, itching, rash.

VALISONE® (Schering Corporation)

Generic Name: Betamethasone valerate

Dosage Form	Strength	Route
Cream	.01%*	Topical (all forms
	.1 %	are applied
Ointment	.1 %	directly
Lotion	.1 %	to affected area)

When Prescribed: Valisone is a potent steroidal drug which is prescribed for the relief of pain, itching and inflammation caused by conditions such as allergic reactions.

Precautions and Warnings: Not for use in the eyes. Valisone should not be used extensively or for prolonged periods in pregnant women.

Side Effects and Adverse Reactions: Burning, itching, irritation, dryness, hair follicle infection, hair growth, pimples, loss of skin color, skin decay, infection.

VALIUM® (Roche Laboratories)

Generic Name: Diazepam

Dosage Form	Strength	Route
Tablet	2 mg*	Oral
	5 mg*	Oral
	10 mg	Oral

When Prescribed: Valium is prescribed for a wide variety of problems to provide relief from tension and anxiety. It is used in a wide variety of physical and/or psychological disorders. It is often prescribed along with other drugs for the relief of muscle or skeletal disorders or for the prevention of convulsions. It is helpful in preventing reactions during withdrawal in alcoholics.

Precautions and Warnings: Patients taking this drug should not drive or operate machinery. Valium should not be taken with alcohol, sedatives, tranquilizers or sleeping pills. A physical and/or psychological dependence on Valium can occur. The use of Valium during pregnancy should almost always be avoided.

Side Effects and Adverse Reactions: Drowsiness, fatigue, loss of balance, confusion, constipation, depression, double vision, aches in joints, fainting, frequent urination, yellowing of skin or eyes, changes in sex drive, nausea, changes in salivation, skin rash, slurred speech, tremors, lack of urination, dizziness, blurred vision, anxiety, hallucinations, muscle spasticity, insomnia, rage, sleep disturbances.

VASODILAN® (Mead Johnson Laboratories)

Generic Name: Isoxsuprine hydrochloride

Dosage Form	Strength	Route
Tablet	10 mg*	Oral
	20 mg	Oral

When Prescribed: Vasodilan is a drug which can increase blood flow to certain areas of the body. It is prescribed for stroke victims, those with cardiovascular diseases and in certain other conditions in which reduced blood flow is present.

Precautions and Warnings: Vasodilan is a potent drug which should only be used under strict control by your physician.

Side Effects and Adverse Reactions: Rash, dizziness, irregular heart beat, nausea, vomiting, abdominal distress.

V–CILLIN K® (Eli Lilly and Company)

Generic Name: Potassium phenoxymethyl penicillin

Dosage Form	Strength	Route
Liquid	125 mg/5 cc	Oral
	250 mg/5 cc*	Oral
Tablet	125 mg	Oral
	250 mg*	Oral
	500 mg	Oral

When Prescribed: V–Cillin K is a form of penicillin which is prescribed for the treatment of mild to moderately severe infections.

Precautions and Warnings: The use of any penicillin should be discontinued and a physician consulted if any of the symptoms listed below appear.

Side Effects and Adverse Reactions: Nausea, vomiting, chest or stomach pains, diarrhea, changes in color/texture of oral membranes, skin rash, hives, chills, fever, swelling, pain in joints, fainting, super-infection by non-susceptible organisms.

VIBRAMYCIN® (Pfizer Laboratories Division)

Generic Name: Doxycycline hyclate

Dosage Form	Strength	Route
Capsule	50 mg	Oral
	100 mg*	Oral
Liquid	25 mg/5 ml	Oral
Liquid	50 mg/5 ml	Oral

When Prescribed: Vibramycin is derived from tetracycline and is an antibiotic prescribed for a variety of infections.

Precautions and Warnings: Vibramycin should not be taken by people overly sensitive to tetracycline. If any of the side effects listed below occur, consult your physician immediately. This drug should not be taken by pregnant women, infants, or children under 8.

Side Effects and Adverse Reactions: Exaggerated sunburn, super-infection by nonsusceptible organisms, loss of appetite, nausea, vomiting, diarrhea, inflammation of the tongue, difficulty swallowing, stomach pains, inflammation of the bowel and genital region, skin rash, hives, swelling, fainting.

VIOFORM-HYDROCORTISONE®
(Ciba Pharmaceutical Company)

Generic Name: Iodochlorhydroxyquin, hydrocortisone

Dosage Form	Strength	Route
Cream	All forms available in one strength only*	Topical (all forms are applied directly to affected area)
Lotion		
Mild cream		
Mild ointment		

When Prescribed: Vioform-hydrocortisone is prescribed for a wide variety of skin disorders.

Precautions and Warnings: This product is not for use in the eye. Vioform-hydrocortisone should not be used extensively by pregnant women in large amounts or for prolonged periods of time.

Side Effects and Adverse Reactions: Rash, sensitivity, local burning, irritation, itching, excessive hair growth, skin infection, hair follicle infection, loss of skin.

VISTARIL® (Pfizer Laboratories Division)

Generic Name: Hydroxyzine pamoate

Dosage Form	Strength	Route
Capsule	25 mg	Oral
	50 mg	Oral
	100 mg	Oral
Liquid	25 mg/5 ml	Oral

When Prescribed: Vistaril is an antihistamine prescribed for the relief of anxiety and tension which can result from a wide variety of emotional or physical reasons. Vistaril is well tolerated by most individuals; for this reason it is often prescribed for long-term use. Also used to prevent vomiting.

Precautions and Warnings: This drug is not recommended for use during early pregnancy. Vistaril should not be taken with alcohol, sleeping pills, sedatives, or tranquilizers unless directed by your physician. If drowsiness occurs you should not drive or operate dangerous machinery. Mothers should not nurse while taking Vistaril.

Side Effects and Adverse Reactions: Drowsiness, dryness of the mouth, tremors, convulsions.

ZAROXOLYN (Pennwalt)

Generic Name: Metolazone

Dosage Form	Strength	Route
Tablet	2.5 mg	Oral
	5 mg	Oral
	10 mg	Oral

When Prescribed: Zaroxolyn is prescribed for the treatment of high blood pressure and for the treatment of water and salt retention resulting from congestive heart failure or kidney disease. It acts by helping the body to pass salt and water.

Precautions and Warnings: This drug should not be taken by nursing mothers.

Side Effects and Adverse Reactions: Constipation, fainting, dizziness, drowsiness, dryness of the mouth, fatigue, muscle weakness, cramps, weakness, restlessness, nausea, vomiting, loss of appetite, diarrhea, bloating, heartburn, yellowing of skin, loss of balance, headache, skin rash, hives, chest pains, chills, yellow appearance of or halo around objects, increased sensitivity to sunlight.

ZYLOPRIM® (Burroughs Wellcome Company)

Generic Name: Allopurinol

Dosage Form	Strength	Route
Tablet	100 mg*	Oral
	300 mg	Oral

When Prescribed: Zyloprim is a potent drug prescribed for the treatment of gout and various related disorders including certain kinds of kidney stones. It is also prescribed for prevention of uric-acid-related syndromes in patients receiving chemotherapy for cancer.

Precautions and Warnings: Zyloprim is a potent drug which should be taken only under close supervision of your physician. Drowsiness can occur. Patients should not drive or operate machinery. This drug should not be taken by nursing mothers. Zyloprim should be discontinued and your physician notified if any of the adverse reactions listed below occurs.

Side Effects and Adverse Reactions: Skin rash, skin eruptions, fever, loss of hair, nausea, vomiting, diarrhea, abdominal pain, chills, itching, drowsiness.

CLASSIFICATION OF DRUGS

ANALGESICS
Darvocet-N   39
Darvon   40
Darvon Compound   40
Darvon-N   41
Demerol   42
Empirin with Codeine   51
Fiorinal   57
Fiorinal with Codeine   58
Percodan   99
Phenaphen with Codeine No. 3   101
Propoxyphene HCl   110
Propoxyphene HCl Compound   111
Pyridium   112
Robaxisal   115
Singlet   120
Soma Compound   121
Synalgos-DC   124
Tabloid® brand A.P.C. with
    Codeine   125
Talwin   126
Tylenol with Codeine   137

ANOREXICS (Diet Pills)
Fastin   56
Ionamin   66
Preludin Endurets   107
Tenuate Dospan   128

ANTIARTHRITICS (Arthritis, Gout)
Benemid   27
Butazolidin   30
Butazolidin Alka   30
Clinoril   34
Indocin   66
Motrin   80
Nalfon   83
Naprosyn   83
Tandearil   127
Tolectin   133
Zyloprim   141

ANTIASTHMATIC, BRONCHODILATOR
Atarax   22
Brethine   29
Choledyl   33
Elixophyllin   51
Isuprel Mistometer   68
Marax   76
Quibron   112
Tedral   127

ANTIBACTERIALS, ANTISEPTICS
AVC Cream   24
Azo Gantanol   24
Azo Gantrisin   25
Bactrim DS   25
Flagyl   58
Gantanol   59
Gantrisin   60
Garamycin Cream   60
Gyne-Lotrimin   61
Lotrimin   75
Macrodantin   75
Mandelamine   76
Monistat 7   80
Mycostatin   81
Septra   118
Sultrin   123
Vioform-Hydrocortisone   140

ANTIBIOTICS (General)
Achromycin V   13
Amcill   17
Amoxicillin   18
Amoxil   18
Ampicillin   19
Bactrim DS   25
Cleocin HCl   34
Declomycin   42
E.E.S.   50
E-Mycin   52
Erythrocin   54
Erythromycin   54
Ilosone   65
Keflex   68
Larotid   71
Minocin   79
Mycolog   81
Mysteclin F   82
Omnipen   91
Panmycin   94
Pediamycin   97
Penicillin G Potassium   97
Penicillin V Potassium   98
Pentids   98
Pen-Vee K   99
Polycillin   105
Principen   108
Robitet   116
Septra   118
Sumycin   123
Terramycin   129
Tetracycline   129
Tetracyn   130
Tetrex   130
V-Cillin K   139
Vibramycin   139

143

INDEX OF DRUGS

NOTES

NOTES

NOTES

NOTES

NOTES

NOTES

NOTES

NOTES

NOTES

NOTES

NOTES

NOTES